DIET METRICS

Hand Book Of Food Exchanges

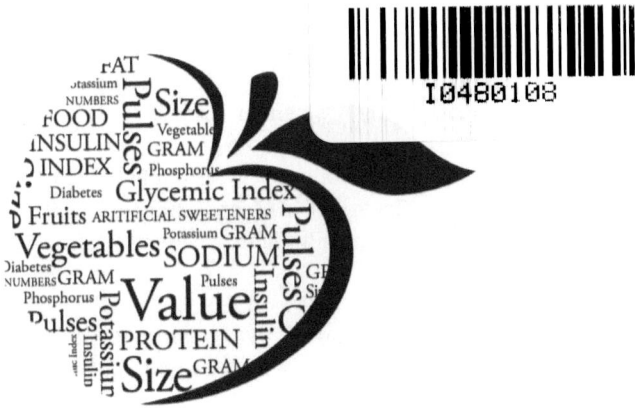

MEENAKSHI BAJAJ

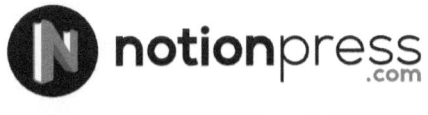

notionpress
.com

INDIA · SINGAPORE · MALAYSIA

Notion Press

Old No. 38, New No. 6
McNichols Road, Chetpet
Chennai - 600 031

First Published by Notion Press 2019
Copyright © Meenakshi Bajaj 2019
All Rights Reserved.

ISBN
Domestic: 978-1-68466-226-5
International: 978-1-64850-636-9

Food Insulin Index

SATIETY   Cereals   GL   Sodium

Fat Protein Unit

Food Exchange list

FEL

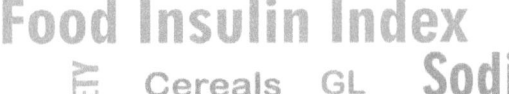

DiET Metrics

Handbook of FoodExchanges

Phosphorus   Exchange

Size

Renal Exchange list

Glycemic Index   GI

Index

Diabetes   DASH   Insulin   CKD

Artificial Sweetners

Diet

Value   Potassium   SALT

FPU   Fruits

Glycemic Load

Numbers   FAT   Vegetables   Gram

Protein   Processed Foods

Carbohydrate   Counting

Unit   Pulses

BI 1st Edition 2019

MEENAKSHI BAJAJ

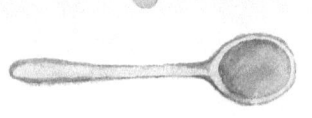

CONTENTS

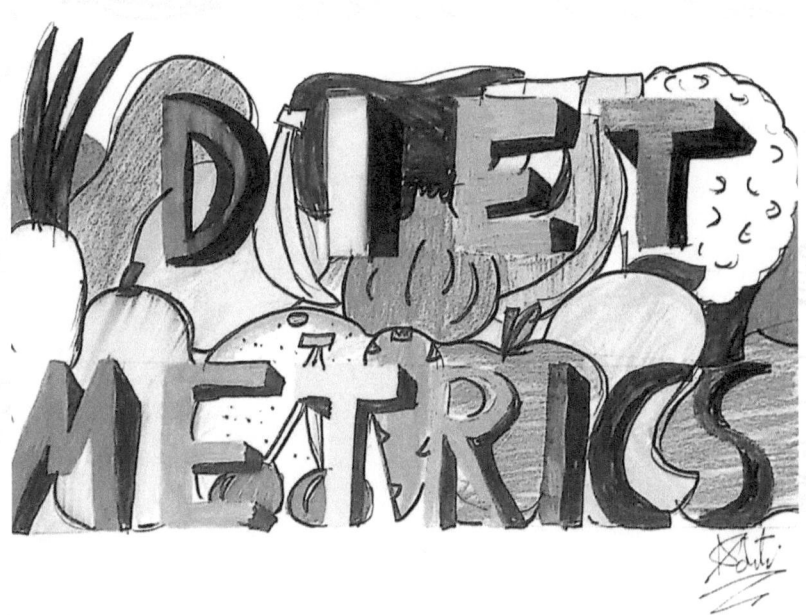

SUPPORTING TEAM

Varsha

Anjali Radhakrishnan

Menaka Srinivasan

Monica V Kothari

Sharon Rebecca

Sonali Kothari

Greata Sherene

Sabiha Begam

Noorul Fahmitha

M.Vijayalakshmi

Monisha Venkatesh

Pavithraa G

Bondhala Lavanya

Goddumarri Mounika

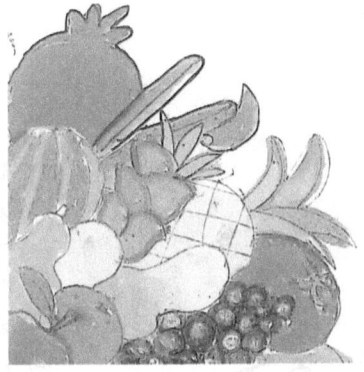

Art by Aditi Lakshmi Bajaj

REVIEWERS

Dr. Nirmala Jesudason PhD, RD. (Academy of Nutrition and Dietetics, USA), Consultant Dietitian and Former RD Board, Chairperson,IDA
Chennai

Dr. Avanti Prabhakhar PG. Diploma in Dietetics, M.Sc., M.Phil., Ph.D., RD
Assistant Professor in Dept. of PG Studies and Research in Home Science
Justice Basheer Ahmed Sayeed College for Women,
Chennai

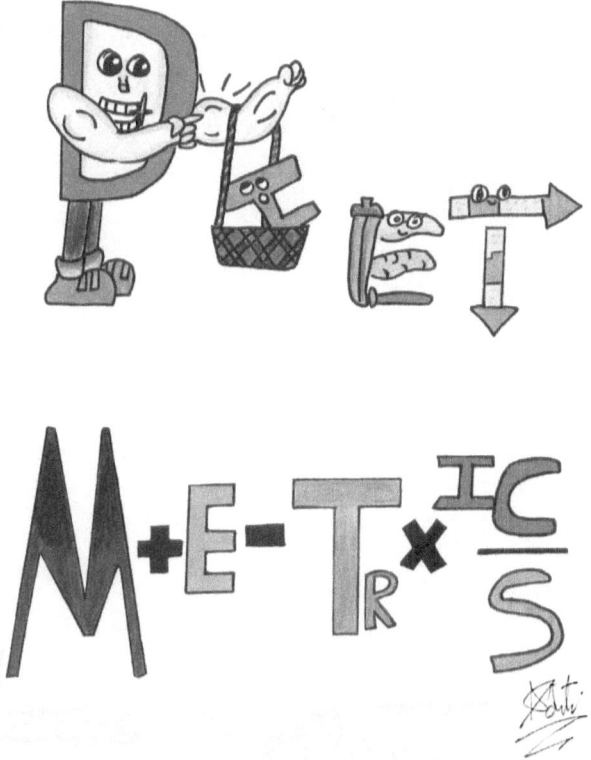

Dr. J. RADHAKRISHNAN, I.A.S.,
Principal Secretary to Government,
Health and Family Welfare Department
Government of Tamil Nadu

Secretariat,
Chennai - 600 009.

Phone : 91-44-2567 1875
Fax   : 91-44-2567 1253
E-Mail : hfwsec@gmail.com

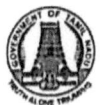

Dated: 24/06/2018

MESSAGE

I am indeed honoured and privileged to convey my message for "DIET METRICS". The recent report on the Global disease burden has highlighted the need to focus on non communicable diseases and the challenges are there for all to see. Lifestyle changes and diet should be the first target when we focus on preventing and also controlling diabetes, blood pressure, obesity and nutrition related challenges.

It is estimated that presently, 95 per cent of all chronic diseases are caused by improper food choice, toxic food ingredients, nutritional deficiencies, and lack of physical exercise. Nutritional management is one of the best non-pharmacological therapies that sometimes is the only remedy or is found to be a valuable and supportive adjuvant to other therapies. One, who neglects nutrition, neglects the skill of a physician. It is in this background that this book assumes importance and relevance and is a unique attempt to put in one place the essential details for deciding on the choices and varieties.

The content and quality of details presented are the result of the author's extensive practical experience and knowledge of

Clinical and Therapeutic Nutrition which has been translated into a comparative study of various food exchanges. The contents of this volume are easy to use, and even easier to apply in real life. I am positive that "DIET METRICS" will act as a key tool for all the dieticians, healthcare professionals, as well as, individuals interested in gaining thorough knowledge on nutritional values for the prevention and management of diabetes, renal and cardio-vascular diseases. With India as the fastest emerging Diabetic Capital of the World, I personally feel this book is going to help the society at large, but most particularly in India. It is being served at the right time by a qualified professional, Ms. Meenakshi Bajaj whose vast experience in Therapeutic Dietetics has proved to be beneficial to several patients in Tamil Nadu Government Hospitals. I have personally witnessed her contribution in revolutionizing the approach in providing disease specific diets in the Omandurar Super specialty hospital which has received appreciation from all who have visited the hospital including those from other States and especially what is extremely heartwarming is that it has received the appreciation of the patients and the caregivers.

My prayers and best wishes to Ms. Bajaj and her team for their dedicated and untiring efforts in this knowledge-sharing endeavour.

DR.J.RADHAKRISHNAN

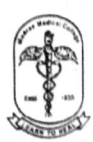

INSTITUTE OF DIABETOLOGY
MADRAS MEDICAL COLLEGE &
RAJIV GANDHI GOVERNMENT GENERAL HOSPITAL
CHENNAI - 600 003. INDIA

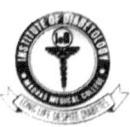

Dr. P. DHARMARAJAN, M.D., D. Diab.,
Professor and Head, Institute of Diabetology,

MESSAGE FROM THE DIABETOLOGIST'S DESK

It is with great pride and pleasure that I attempt to write this message on the occasion of the publication of the book on nutrition by Mrs. Meenakshi Bajaj. This book on nutrition aims at improving the practical knowledge of all the physicians and stakeholders practicing in the field of diabetes and endocrinology. I strongly believe that this improvement of practical knowledge in nutrition and dietetics which forms an integral and vital part of managing any patient with diabetes will definitely go a long way to help improve the standards of care of patients with diabetes which is being practiced as on date. The simple language and terms of references pertaining to locally available foodstuffs and nutritional products will, for sure, help to clear the doubts and ambiguities on the minds of all the medical practitioners, dieticians, nutritionists, paramedical workers, students and all those involved in the care of patients with diabetes mellitus. This will, in turn, translate into better care of patients with diabetes, which is indeed the need of the hour, as far as our country is concerned.

I wish the book and its author the best of success in all future endeavors.

Dr. P. DHARMARAJAN
Professor and Head, Institute of Diabetology,
Madras Medical College and
Rajiv Gandhi Government General Hospital, Chennai.

MESSAGE FROM THE NEPHROLOGIST'S DESK

Dr. S. Jayalakshmi

It gives me immense pleasure to write a message for this scholarly publication on nutrient exchanges. This book is a practical guide for Doctors and Allied health care professionals associated with nutrition management. The detailed account of the composition of various indigenous food products will be of great help in guiding the healthcare professionals to modify the dietary pattern of the patient whenever necessary. The simple language and the user-friendly approach will be of great benefit to the readers. The author of this book, Ms. Meenakshi Bajaj is a dedicated Nutritionist whose foremost priority is patient wellness. My best wishes to her on this endeavor.

Jayalakshmi

Dr. S. JAYALAKSHMI D.C.H., M.D. (Gen.Med), D.M. (Nephro)
Senior Consultant and Professor of Nephrology,
TamilNadu Government Multi Super Specialty Hospital,
Omandurar Estate, Chennai 600002.

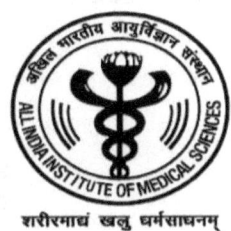

अखिल भारतीय आयुर्विज्ञान संस्थान

अंसारी नगर, नई दिल्ली-110029

ALL INDIA INSTITITE OF MEDICAL SCIENCES

ANSARI NAGAR, NEW DELHI-110029

शरीरमाद्यं खलु धर्मसाधनम्   दिनांक/Dated: 18-04-2018

MESSAGE

I am indeed privileged to share the message for Ms. Meenakshi Bajaj, on her step towards the making of the pocket guide 'DIET METRICS'.

This book allows easy access to essential nutritional information. I take the opportunity to congratulate the collaborative efforts of her team for taking up this venture with commitment in the interest and welfare of the patients.

I believe this volume belongs on the bookshelf of every health care provider who deals with patients with diabetes or renal complications.

The content has been culled from authentic sources to provide nutrient data in a nutshell. Thus "DIET METRICS" is an evidence-based reference for health care professionals to calculate with ease and convenience during their clinical practice.

Wishing the team of supporting team many more editions

(Dr. ALKA MOHAN CHUTANI)

Chief Dietician & Head

Department of Dietetics

AIIMS, New Delhi.

FOREWORD

Medical Nutrition Therapy is a powerful clinical and therapeutic tool in the prevention, management, and treatment of various diseases. Several nutrition tools are utilized for effective menu planning and "DIET METRICS" proves to be a good step in this direction.

The book "DIET METRICS" is written by a senior practicing dietitian Ms. Meenakshi Bajaj, with extensive knowledge and over 25 years of experience in the field of Clinical Nutrition and Dietetics. I am honored to write a few lines about this comprehensive guide on various food exchanges.

The primary objective of this book is to provide accurate and current scientific information with regard to easy access to nutrient contents for quick and effective menu planning, which is the need of the hour. It not only presents nutrition facts but also helps the reader to apply these facts into clinical practice.

The author along with her team has painstakingly brought out this comprehensive book which succeeds in providing nutritional information that is relevant to practicing dietitians, academicians, diabetologists, nephrologists, nutrition and nursing students, research scholars, cookery experts, and entrepreneurs. I am confident that this book will be an asset to the field of Clinical Nutrition and Dietetics.

It is necessary to equip both professionals and students of Nutrition and Dietetics with state-of-the-art knowledge and nutrition information on commonly consumed foods. This book will help readers gain valuable insights and help them incorporate foods in customized/ patient specific meal plans in order to meet optimal nutritional needs as well as ensure patient satisfaction.

I highly recommend "DIET METRICS" for the worktable of all healthcare professionals managing Non-communicable diseases as it would serve as a ready reference in the management of various ailments.

Wishing this value-added edition all success!

Dr. SHEILA JOHN MSc, MPhil, PhD
Associate Professor and Head
Department of Home Science,
Women's Christian College,
Chennai-6.

PREFACE

Diet therapy is an important component of Lifestyle Medicine. The major barrier about a diet chart is that it revolves around dietary restrictions and occasionally limited menu options. A standard food exchange system aids in easy menu planning with flexibility, ample food choices and most importantly reminding the Health Care Professional (HCP) to include all food exchange groups in order to meet disease-specific nutrient requirements.

The concept of using Food Exchange Lists traces back to the 1950s by the Academy of Nutrition and Dietetics, USA. Globally each and every dietetic professional need to follow a standard exchange list prepared from recent, validated and nation-specific nutrient database. Having varied food patterns throughout our country we require one Meal Planning Food Exchange List (MPFEL) for basic as well as therapeutic menu planning.

Presently each region in our country is following a different exchange list and a few are not having access to user-friendly exchanges. This motivated me to initiate the exercise to develop "DIET METRICS".

"DIET METRICS" is a user- friendly tool providing an insight on Standard Meal Planning Exchanges, Glycemic friendly and Renal Food Exchanges. Each of these exchanges has been extracted and summed up from the most standardized, recent and validated, Indian Food Composition Table (2017).

However, to ensure that this tool is more effective, nutrition care process details along with cultural variations will have to be taken into consideration. Portion size determination is also a prerequisite to ascertaining the nutrient adequacy of any dietary regime. "DIET METRICS" would prove to be a simple and handy tool to convert the nutrition prescription with near accuracy and ease to a practical menu plan, both at an individual and community level. Medical and allied healthcare professionals may find "DIET METRICS" as a valuable addition to their bookshelf.

In the compilation of these detailed exchanges, errors and omissions are inevitable. Also, scientific techniques are constantly being improved and nutritional theory continues to advance with ongoing researches. I humbly request the readers to point out any inaccuracies for necessary updation in the subsequent editions.

It is my hope and expectation that this book would prove to be a useful reference resource in Therapeutic Dietetics.

Ms. MEENAKSHI BAJAJ PG.D.N.D., M.Sc., RD., CDE., CCN (U.S). (Ph.D.).,
Dietician, Tamil Nadu Government Multi Super Specialty Hospital, Omandurar Estate, Chennai-02.
President, Indian Dietetic Association, Chennai Chapter (2015–18).
National Executive Committee Member, Indian Dietetic Association (2019-2021)
National Executive Committee Member, Association of Diabetes Educators (India)
Former Dietician, Institute of Diabetology, Rajiv Gandhi Government General Hospital, Chennai-03.

ACKNOWLEDGMENTS

I place on record my heartfelt thanks to the National Institute of Nutrition for their valuable contribution "The Indian Food Composition Tables (2017)" without which "DIET METRICS" wouldn't have been possible.

We are greatly indebted to The Principal Secretary, Health and Family Welfare Department, Government of Tamil Nadu, Dr. J.Radhakrishnan I.A.S for his constant encouragement to the Dietetic Fraternity to provide the best in terms of health and nutrition support to the society. I express my gratitude to Sir for sharing his valuable message for "DIET METRICS".

I convey my sincere thanks to Prof. P.Dharmarajan, M.D., D. Diab., from Madras Medical College & Rajiv Gandhi Govt. General Hospital, Prof. S.Jayalakshmi, D.C.H., M.D., D.M (Nephro) from Tamil Nadu Government Multi Super Specialty, Dr. Alka Mohan Chutani Ph.D., (Foods & Nutrition) from All India Institute of Medical Sciences for their valuable message for "DIET METRICS" I owe my sincere thanks to Dr. Nirmala Jesudason and Dr. Avanti Prabhakhar for spending their valuable time in editing and reviewing the book. My wholehearted thanks to Dr.Sheila John, Ph.D., from Women's Christian College, Chennai for her valuable contribution towards "DIET METRICS".

I especially recognize the untiring efforts of all my colleagues for their timely contribution to make this book possible. Support rendered by my interns is remarkable and memorable.

My heartfelt gratitude to my parents and sisters who were the driving source behind the completion of this long-cherished dream of mine. Their encouragement and support take me always to the horizon of my purpose and allow me to look beyond it.

I am deeply indebted to my mentors, Dr.Patricia Trueman, Ms. Srilakshmi .B & Dr. Suganthi Mouli for grooming me to scale great heights in the field of Clinical Nutrition and Dietetics.

I am thankful to Dr. Dharini Krishnan, Ms Salome Benjamin, Prof. R.S. Hariharan, Prof. N. Rajendiran, Prof. D. Shantaram, Prof. Anand Moses & Prof. R. Madhavan Former Director's of The Institute of Diabetology, Rajiv Gandhi Govt. General Hospital, Chennai for being a constant source of inspiration and encouragement.

Special thanks to Mr. M.S. Vasanthan, Ms. Monisha Venkatesh and Ms. Pavithraa Gopinath for their valuable inputs in images, editing, and designing "DIET METRICS".

My heartfelt gratitude to Ms. Ramya Ramachandran for her contribution in coining the title "DIET METRICS".

I find no words that would adequately thank my husband and daughter for giving me space and freedom to pursue my dreams to reality.

Notion Press needs special appreciation and thanks for undertaking the responsibility of support, quality printing and timely completion of the book.

What's Inside?

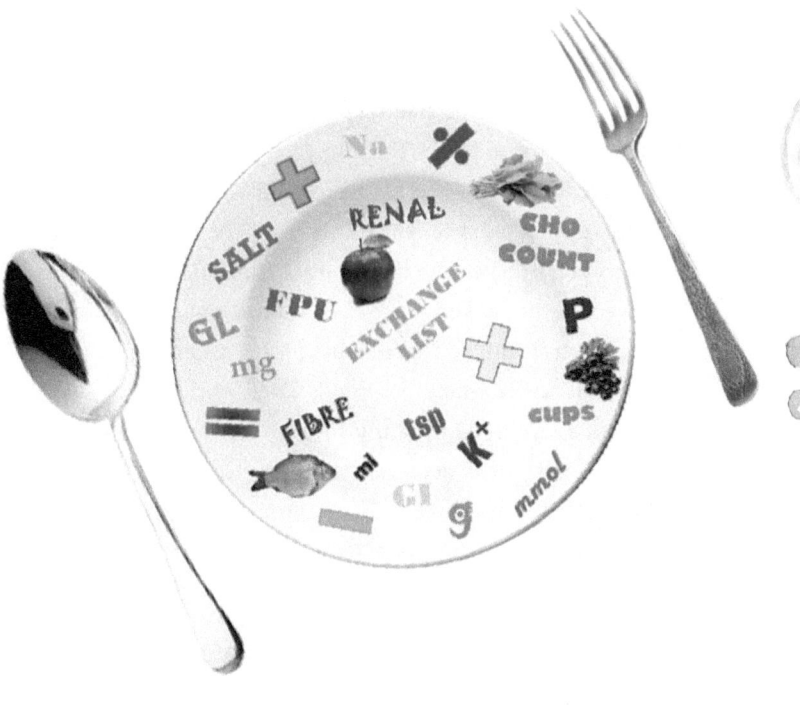

DIET METRICS is a user- friendly tool providing an insight on Standard Meal Planning Exchanges, Glycemic friendly and Renal Food Exchanges. Each of these exchanges have been extracted and summed up from the most standardized, recent and validated, Indian Food Composition Table (2017).

However, to ensure that this tool is more effective, nutrition care process details along with cultural variations will have to be taken into consideration. Portion size determination is also a prerequisite to ascertain nutrient adequacy of any dietary regime.   DIET METRICS would prove to be a simple and handy tool to convert the nutrition prescription with near accuracy and ease to a practical menu plan, both at an individual and community level. Medical and allied health care professionals may find DIET METRICS as a valuable addition to their book shelf.

MEAL PLANNING FOOD EXCHANGE LIST (MPFEL)

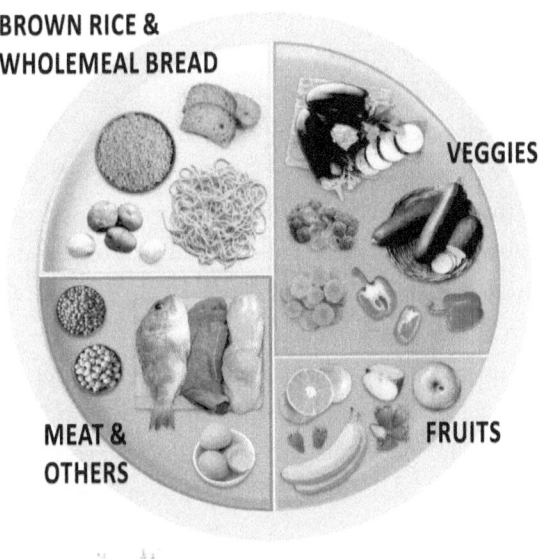

BROWN RICE &
WHOLEMEAL BREAD

VEGGIES

MEAT &
OTHERS

FRUITS

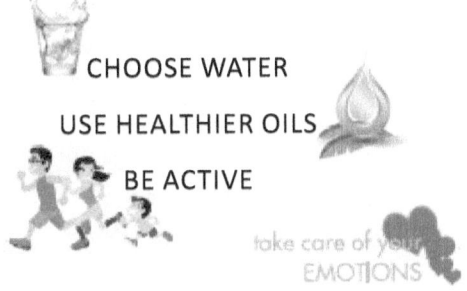

CHOOSE WATER

USE HEALTHIER OILS

BE ACTIVE

take care of your
EMOTIONS

MEAL PLANNING FOOD EXCHANGE LIST

Diet and nutrition are important factors in the promotion and maintenance of good health throughout the entire life and therefore, it occupies a prominent position in preventive medicine (World Health Organisation, 2003).

Exchange lists are foods listed together under different food groups such as cereals, pulses, milk, meat and its products, nuts, fats & oils, fruits and vegetables (Krause's, 2016), where each serving of a food has about the same amount of carbohydrate, protein, fat, and calories as the other foods on that list (Misra, 2011).

Food Exchange List is an appropriate tool for effective nutrition education, intended for improving nutrition knowledge, attitudes and dietary behaviors both at an individual and community level (Love, Maunder, Ross, Lovely & Charlton, 2001). It is also considered to be a practical dietary tool designed to help dieticians to convert diet prescription into a meal plan and also help patients to wisely choose on variety of foods among each food group by maintaining adequate nutrient content and satisfy the requirement of a given individual (Khan, Kalsoom & Khan, 2017; Gopalan, Sastri & Balasubramanian, 2010).

However, to ensure that this tool is more effective cultural variations will have to be taken into consideration so as to provide the user with food items with which he or she is more familiar as exact menus and food amounts are a prerequisite to ascertaining the nutrient adequacy of any dietary regime.

References

1. Gopalan, C., Sastri, B .V. R., & Balasubramanian, S. C. (1989). *Nutritive Value of Indian Foods (Rev.ed.).* India, Hyderabad: National Institute of Nutrition.
2. Khan, M.N., Kalsoom, S. & Khan, A.A. (2017). Food Exchange List and Dietary Management of Non-communicable Disease in Cultural Perspective. *Pakistan Journal of Medical Science, 33*(5), 1273-1278.
3. Love, P., Maunder, E., Ross, F., Lovely, S.J. & Charlton, K. (2001). South African food-based dietary guidelines: testing of the preliminary guidelines among women in KwaZulu-Natal and the Western Cape. *South African Journal of Clinical Nutrition, 14*(1), 9-19.
4. Mahan, L.K., & Raymond, J.L. (Eds.) (2016). *Krause's food & the nutrition care process,* (14ᵗʰ ed.). St.Louis, Missouri: Elsevier.
5. Misra, R. (Ed.) (2011). *Indian Foods: AAPI's Guide to Nutrition, Health, and Diabetes.* Chennai: Allied Publishers Private Limited.
6. World Health Organization. (2003): *Diet, nutrition, and prevention of chronic disease.* Report of a joint FAO and WHO Expert Consultation, Geneva, (2002). WHO Technical Report Series, 916. Geneva: World Health Organization.

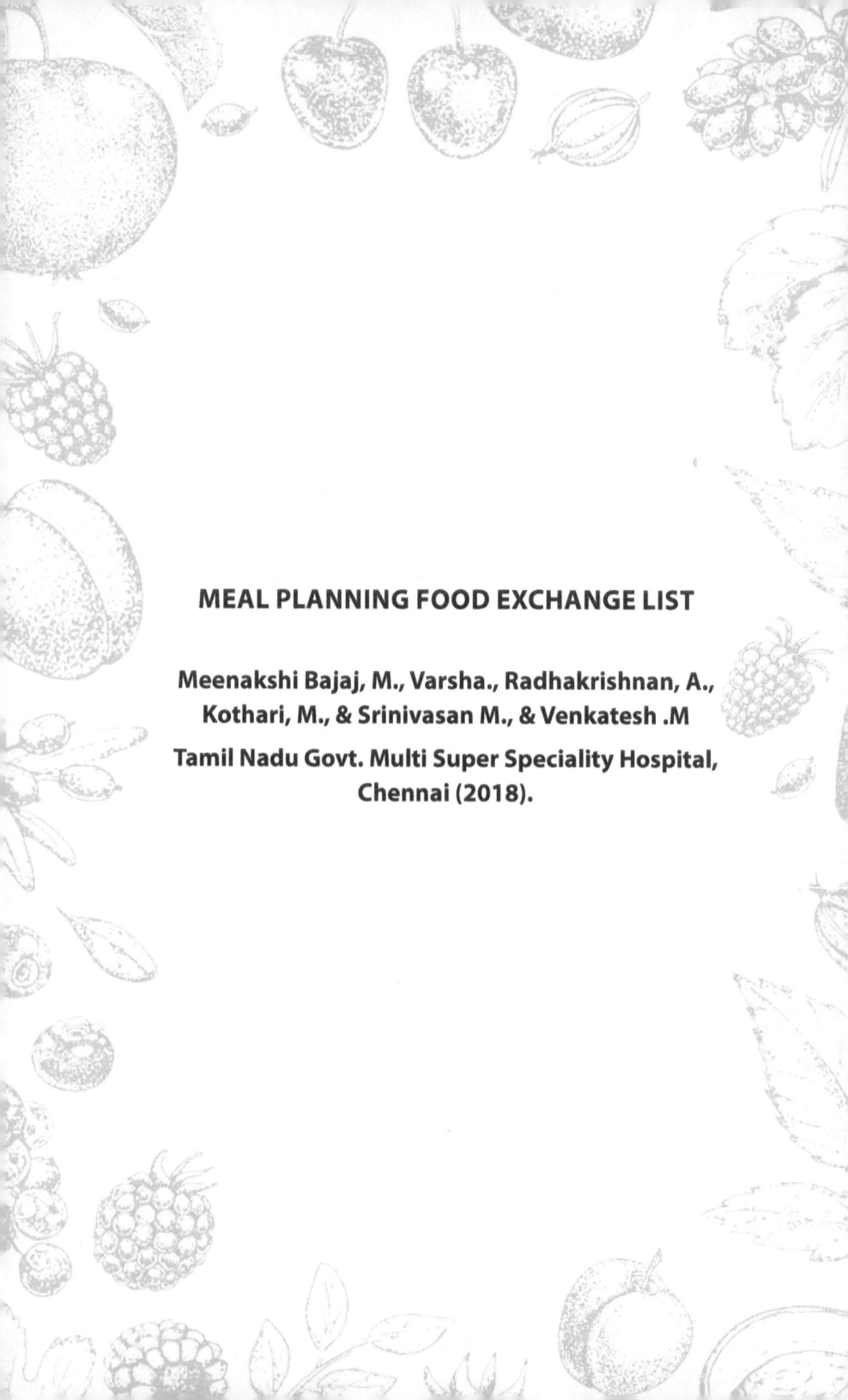

MEAL PLANNING FOOD EXCHANGE LIST

Meenakshi Bajaj, M., Varsha., Radhakrishnan, A., Kothari, M., & Srinivasan M., & Venkatesh .M

Tamil Nadu Govt. Multi Super Speciality Hospital, Chennai (2018).

CEREAL EXCHANGE LIST

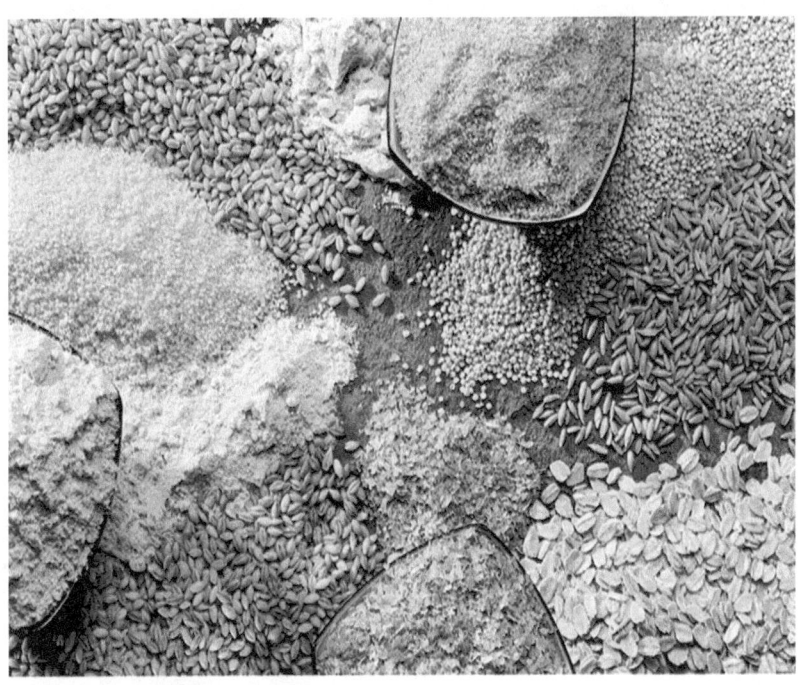

1 CEREAL EXCHANGE	
Energy	80 – 94 kcal
Carbohydrate	13 – 21 g
Protein	1 – 3.5 g
Fat	0 – 2.0 g
Fiber	1 – 4.0 g

Source: IFCT (2017)

Note:

- Energy value mentioned in the above Cereal exchange is an average of the commonly consumed cereals.

1 CEREAL EXCHANGE LIST

Food Ingredient	Raw weight (g)	Cooked portion
Barley	25	1 cup
Cornflakes	25	-
Dosa flour(Dry)	25 (Cereal: Pulse 4:1)	1 medium
Idly flour(Dry)	25 (Cereal: Pulse 4:1)	1 large
Oats	25	-
Quinoa	25	-
Rice flakes(Dry)	25	⅓ cup
Rice, raw milled	25	½ cup
Vermicelli(Dry)	25	½ cup
Wheat, semolina(dry)	25	½ cup
*Whole wheat flour	25	30g (Chapati – 1 No, medium) 6"diameter
Wheat Bread, white	-	25g is one slice

Note:

- * Wheat Bread, white- 1 slice (25g) -10cm width, Thickness- 1cm, Providing 61 kcal/slice

SAGO EXCHANGE

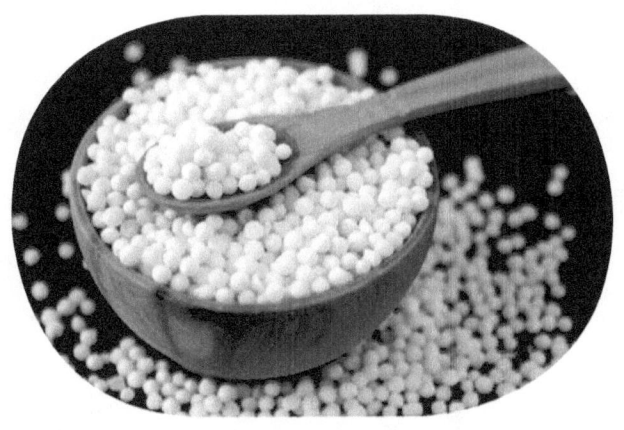

1 SAGO EXCHANGE	
Energy	88 kcal
Carbohydrate	22 g
Protein	Negligible
Fat	Negligible
Fiber	Negligible

1 SAGO EXCHANGE		
Food Ingredient	Raw weight (g)	Cooked portion
Sago*	25	1 cup

Source: IFCT (2017)

MILLET EXCHANGE LIST

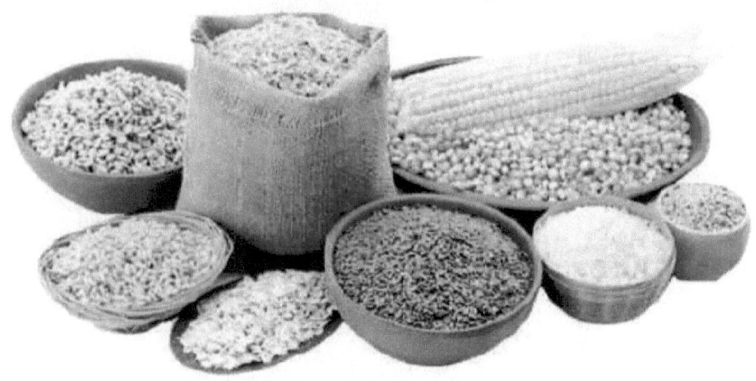

1 MILLET EXCHANGE	
Energy	78 – 87 kcal
Carbohydrate	15.5 – 17.0 g
Protein	2 – 3 g
Fat	0.5 – 1.5 g
Fiber	2 – 3 g

1 MILLET EXCHANGE LIST		
Food Ingredient	**Raw weight (g)**	**Cooked portion**
Pearl Millet/Bajra	25	½ cup
Jowar/Sorghum	25	½ cup
Finger Millet/Ragi	25	½ cup
Little Millet /Samai	25	½ cup
Kodo Millet /Varagu	25	½ cup

Source: IFCT (2017)

Note:

- Energy value mentioned in the above Millet exchange is an average of the energy values of the commonly consumed millets.

PULSE EXCHANGE LIST

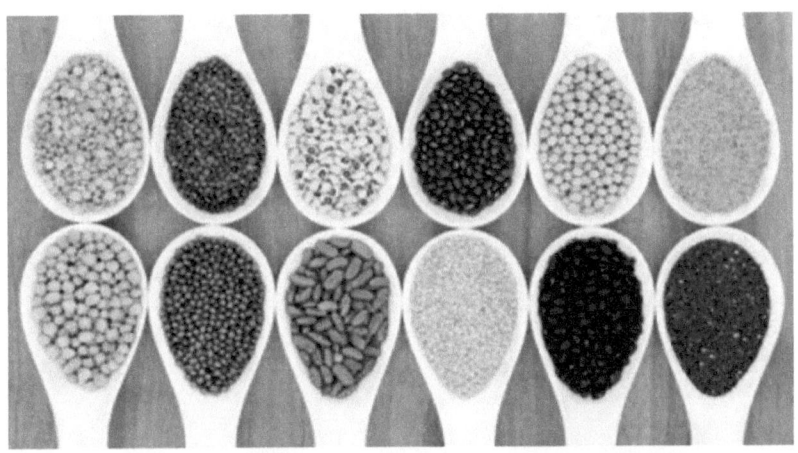

1 PULSE EXCHANGE	
Energy	81 – 83 kcal
Carbohydrate	12.0 – 14.0 g
Protein	5.5 – 6.0 g
Fat	0 – 1.5 g
Fiber	2.0 – 4.0 g

1 PULSE EXCHANGE LIST		
Food Ingredient	**Raw weight (g)**	**Cooked portion**
Bengal gram, dal	25	½ cup
Black gram, dal	25	½ cup
Green gram, dal	25	½ cup
Lentil Dal	25	½ cup
Red gram, dal	25	½ cup

Source: IFCT (2017)

Note:

- Energy value mentioned in the above Pulse exchange is an average of the energy values of the commonly consumed pulses.

WHOLE GRAM EXCHANGE LIST

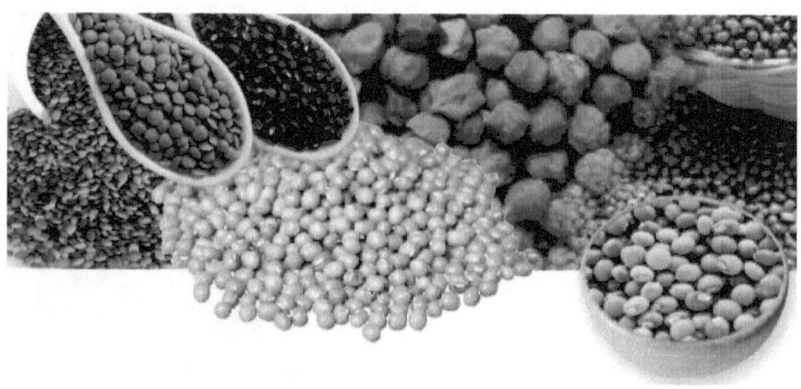

1 WHOLE GRAM EXCHANGE	
Energy	69 – 83 kcal
Carbohydrate	10.0 – 14.5 g
Protein	5.0 – 6.0 g
Fat	0 – 1 g
Fiber	2.0 – 6.5 g

1 WHOLE GRAM EXCHANGE LIST		
Food Ingredient	Raw weight (g)	Cooked portion
Bengal gram, whole	25	½ cup
Black gram, whole	25	½ cup
Green gram, whole	25	½ cup
Horse gram, whole	25	½ cup
Lentil whole, brown	25	½ cup
Red gram, whole	25	½ cup

Source: IFCT (2017)

Note:

- Energy value mentioned in the above Whole gram exchange is an average of the energy values of the commonly consumed whole grams.

SOYABEAN EXCHANGE LIST

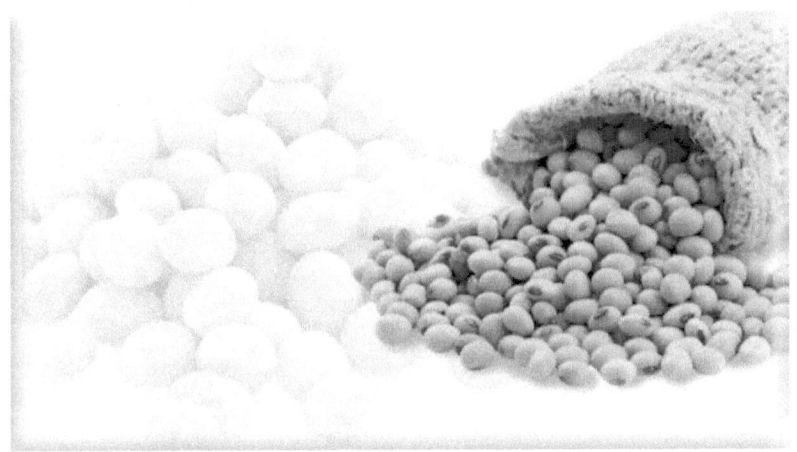

1 SOYA BEAN EXCHANGE	
Energy	75 kcal
Carbohydrate	2.0 g
Protein	8.0 g
Fat	4.0 g
Fiber	4.5 g

1 SOYA BEAN EXCHANGE		
Food Ingredient	Raw weight (g)	Cooked portion
Soya bean	20	½ cup

Source: IFCT (2017)

MILK EXCHANGE LIST

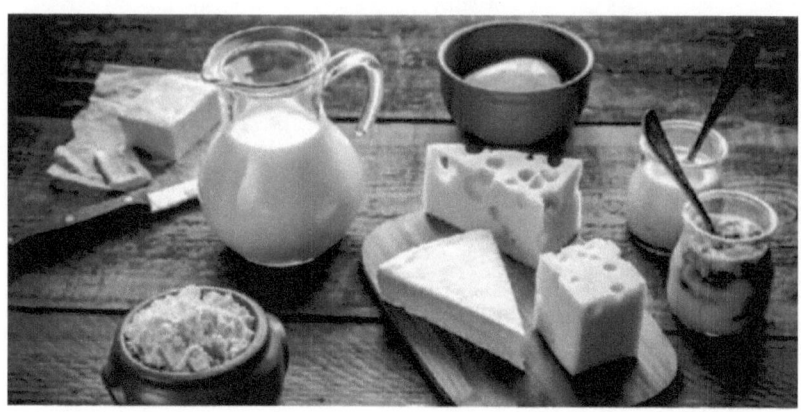

1 MILK EXCHANGE	
Energy	110 Kcal
Carbohydrate	6.0 – 8.5 g
Protein	4.0 – 6.0 g
Fat	6.5 – 7.5 g
Fiber	Negligible

1 MILK EXCHANGE LIST		(1 cup = 200 ml)
Food Ingredient	Raw weight	Portion Size
Buffalo milk	100 ml	½ cup
Cow's milk	150 ml	¾ cup
#Curd (cow's milk)	185 g	<1 cup

Source: IFCT (2017) & #NIN (1989)

1 SKIMMED MILK EXCHANGE	
Energy	100Kcal
Carbohydrate	14.0 – 16.0g
Protein	9.0 – 11.0g
Fat	Negligible
Fiber	0

1 SKIMMED MILK EXCHANGE LIST		
Food Ingredient	Raw weight (g)	Portion Size
*Skimmed milk	350ml	1¾ cup
*Skimmed milk powder	28g	5 ½ tsp

* *Source:* NIN (1989)

Nutritional Information/100g
Fresh Paneer, (Cow's Milk)

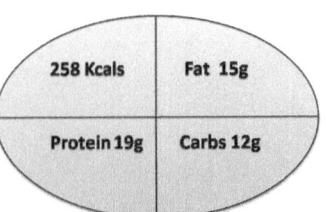

258 Kcals	Fat 15g
Protein 19g	Carbs 12g

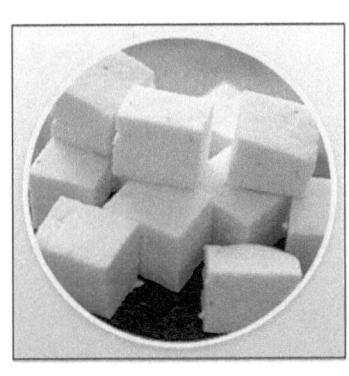

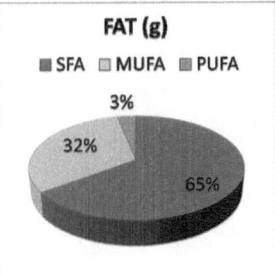

FAT (g)

■ SFA ▨ MUFA ■ PUFA

3%

32%

65%

MEAT, POULTRY, AND MARINE
EXCHANGE LIST

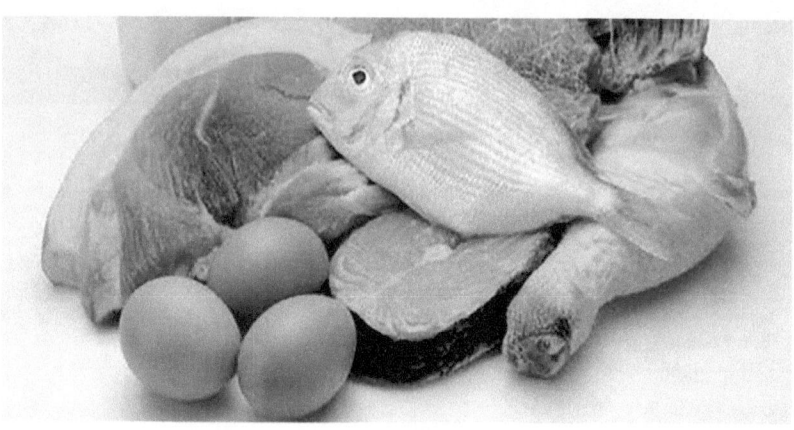

1 MEAT EXCHANGE	
Energy	84 – 91 kcal
Carbohydrate	Negligible
Protein	11.0 – 13.0 g
Fat	4.0 – 5.0 g
Fiber	Negligible

1 MEAT EXCHANGE LIST		
Food Ingredient	Raw Weight (g)	Cooked portion
Beef, Chops	65	-
Chicken, poultry, breast, skinless	50	-
Goat, Chops	65	-

Source: IFCT (2017)

EGG EXCHANGE LIST

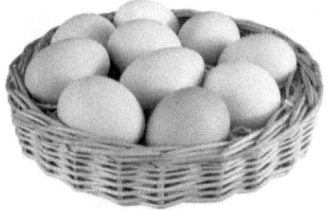

1 EGG	50g
Egg yolk	15g
Egg white	30g
Shell	5g

1 EGG EXCHANGE		
Food Ingredient	Raw Weight (g)	Quantity
Egg, poultry, whole, raw	50	1 no

NUTRITIONAL INFORMATION ON AN EGG		
Food Ingredient Egg, poultry, raw (50g)	Egg White (30 g)	Egg Yolk (15 g)
Energy (Kcal)	13.4	44.57
Protein (g)	3.25	2.36
Fat (g)	Negligible	3.95

1 EGG EXCHANGE	
Energy	67 kcal
Carbohydrate	Negligible
Protein	6.6 g
Fat	4.6 g
Fiber	Negligible

Source: IFCT (2017)

MARINE FOODS EXCHANGE LIST

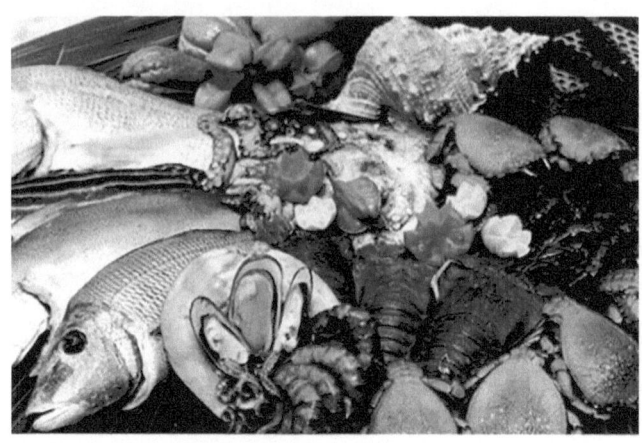

1 MARINE FOODS EXCHANGE	
Energy	85 kcal
Carbohydrate	Negligible
Protein	13.0 – 19.0g
Fat	1.0 – 3.0 g
Fiber	Negligible

1 MARINE FOODS EXCHANGE LIST		
Food Ingredient	Raw weight (g)	Cooked portion
Crab, sea	125	-
Mackerel	85	-
Pomphret, black	69	-
Prawn, small	120	-
Tuna	76	-

Source: IFCT (2017)

GROUP A (GREEN LEAFY) VEGETABLES EXCHANGE

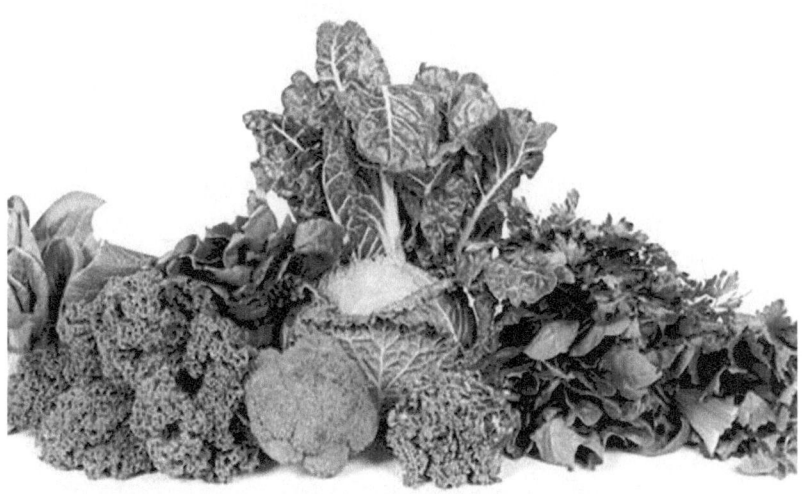

GROUP A (GREEN LEAFY) VEGETABLES EXCHANGE	
Energy	34–36 kcal
Carbohydrate	2.0–5.0 g
Protein	2.5–4.5 g
Fat	≤ 1.0 g
Fiber	2.5–5.0 g
*Fibre	9.0 g

GROUP A (LEAFY VEGETABLES) EXCHANGE LIST		
Food Ingredient	Raw weight (g)	Cooked portion
Agathi leaves	50	¼ cup
Amaranth leaves	115	½ cup
Cabbage green	160	¾ cup
Cauliflower leaves	100	½ cup
Coriander leaves	110	½ cup
*Curry leaves	55	¼ cup
Drumstick leaves	50	¼ cup
Fenugreek leaves	100	½ cup
Lettuce	160	¾ cup
Mint	95	½ cup
Mustard leaves	115	½ cup
Ponnanganni	70	¾ cup
Radish leaves	135	¾ cup
Spinach	145	¾ cup

Source: IFCT (2017)

*Curry Leaves

GROUP B (ROOTS & TUBERS) EXCHANGE LIST

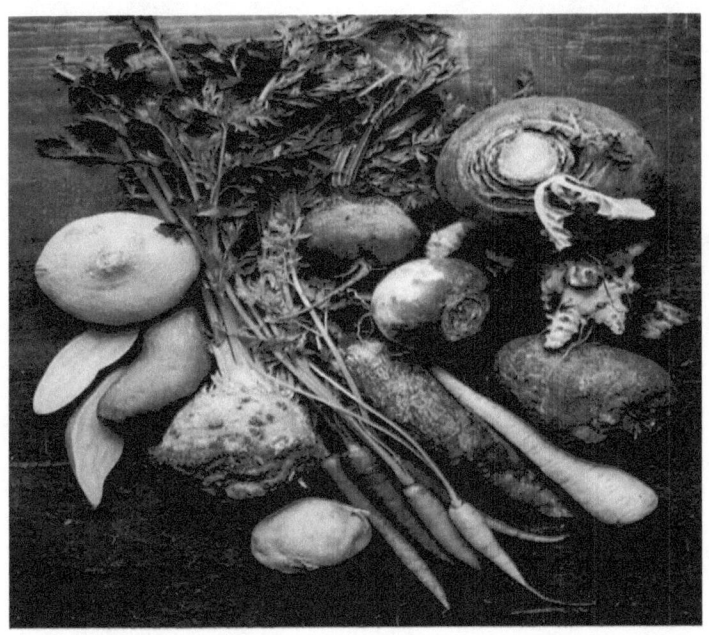

GROUP B VEGETABLES (ROOTS AND TUBERS) EXCHANGE	
Energy	48–54 kcal
Carbohydrate	8.0–12.0 g
Protein	0.5–3.0 g
Fat	≤1 g
Fiber	1.0–6.5 g

GROUP B (ROOTS AND TUBERS) EXCHANGE LIST

Food Ingredient	Raw weight (g)	Cooked portion
Beetroot	140	¾ cup
Carrot, orange	150	¾ cup
Carrot, red	130	¾ cup
Colocasia	55	¼ cup
Onion, big	100	½ cup
Potato, brown skin big	75	<½ cup
Sweet potato, pink skin	50	<½ cup
Radish, round, white skin	160	<¾ cup
Tapioca	65	<½ cup
Yam	60	<½ cup

Source: IFCT (2017)

Note:

• Tubers are least in fiber

GROUP C (OTHER VEGETABLES) EXCHANGE LIST

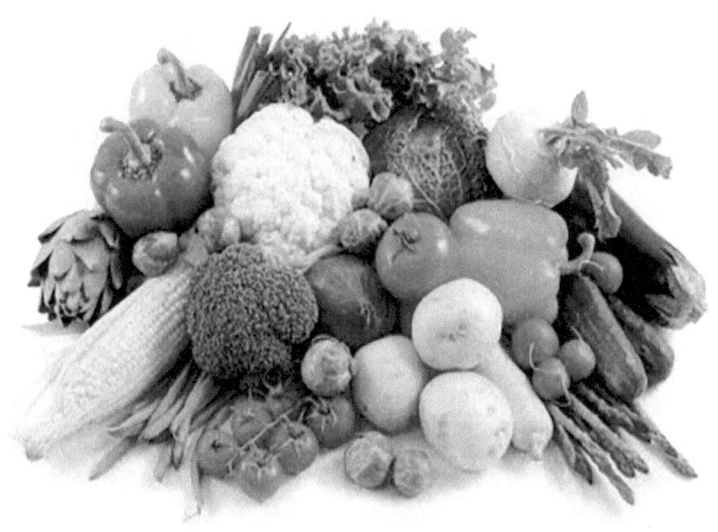

GROUP C (OTHER VEGETABLES) EXCHANGE	
Energy	28–30 kcal
Carbohydrate	2.0–6.0 g
Protein	0.5–4.0 g
Fat	≤ 1.0 g
Fiber	1.5–7.5 g

Source: IFCT (2017)

Note:

- Drumstick & Bean varieties contain 3-4 g protein
- Drumstick, Gourd & Bean varieties contain>5 g fiber

GROUP C (OTHER VEGETABLES) EXCHANGE LIST

Food Ingredient	Raw weight (g)	Cooked portion
Ash gourd	170	¾ cup
Beans scarlet, tender	70	<½ cup
Bitter gourd, jagged, teeth ridges, elongate	145	¾ cup
Bottle gourd, elongate, pale green	270	1½ cup
Brinjal all varieties	120	½ cup
Broad beans	100	½ cup
Capsicum, green	185	<1 cup
Cauliflower	130	>½ cup
Cho- Cho-marrow	160	¾ cup
Corn, Baby	40	<½ cup
Cucumber, green, elongate	150	¾ cup
Drumstick	100	<½ cup
French beans, Country	125	½ cup
Knol-Khol	190	¾ cup
Kovai, big	170	¾ cup
Ladies finger	110	<½ cup
Mango, green, raw	60	<½ cup
Parwar	125	<½ cup
Plantain flower	140	<½ cup
Plantain, green	35	<½ cup
Plantain, stem	75	<½ cup
Pumpkin, green, cylindrical	120	½ cup
Pumpkin, orange, round	130	½ cup
Ridge gourd	230	2 cup
Snake gourd, long, pale green	240	<2½ cup
Tinda, tender	200	1 cup
Tomato, green	220	¾ cup
Tomato, ripe, hybrid	160	<1½ cup
Tomato, ripe, local	155	<1½ cup
Zucchini, green	150	¾ cup

NUT EXCHANGE LIST

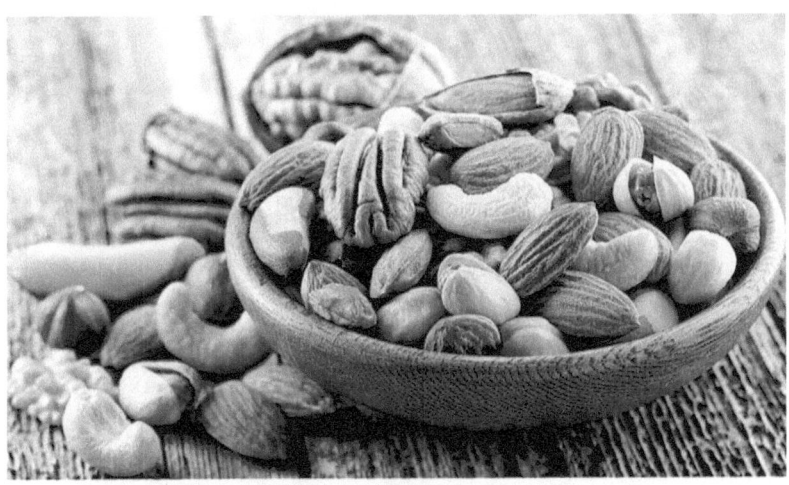

1 NUT EXCHANGE	
Energy	83–87 kcal
Carbohydrate	4 g
Protein	4 g
Fat	6.0–9.0 g
Fiber	1–2 g

1 NUT EXCHANGE LIST		
Food Ingredient	Raw weight (g)	Quantity
Almond	14.0	12 no
Cashew	14.5	6 no
Coconut, kernel, fresh	21.0	4 Tsp
Groundnut	16.0	20 no
Pistachio	16.0	24 no
Walnut	13.0	5 no

Source: IFCT (2017)

FRUIT EXCHANGE LIST

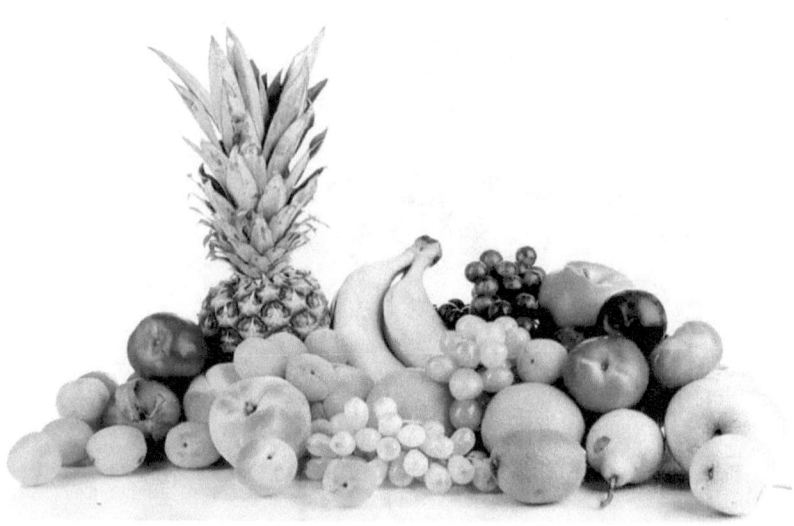

1 FRUIT EXCHANGE LIST	
Energy	40 kcal
Carbohydrate	6.0–9.5 g
Protein	0.5–1.5 g
Fat	≤ 1 g#
Fiber	1.0–5.5 g

Source: IFCT (2017)

Note

- #Avocado contains 4 g of fat /exchange
- Guava contains >5g of fiber/ exchange

1 FRUIT EXCHANGE LIST

Food Ingredients	Raw weight (g)	Rounded off to nearest whole no Raw weight (g)	Quantity
Apple, big	64	70	1/2 Big
Apricot, dried	13	15	-
Avocado fruit	27	25	-
Banana, poovam	38	40	1/2 Medium
Banana, ripe, red	36	40	-
Cherries, red	67	70	-
Custard apple	41	40	1 Medium
Dates, processed	14	15	2 no
Fig	50	50	-
Gooseberry	170	170	-
Grapes, seeded, round, green	72	75	18-20 no
Grapes, seeded, round, black	66	70	-
Guava, pink flesh	86	90	-
Guava, white flesh	124	125	1 Medium
Jackfruit, ripe	56	50	3 no
Jambu fruit, ripe	72	70	12 no
Lime, sweet pulp	148	150	-
Litchi	75	75	-
Muskmelon, orange flesh	173	175	4-5 slices
Orange Pulp	108	110	1 Medium
Papaya, ripe	168	170	4 Thin long slices
Pear	107	110	1 Medium
Pineapple	93	100	1 Thick Slice
Plum	71	70	5 no
Sapota	55	60	1/2 Big
Strawberry	164	170	-
Tamarind, pulp	14	15	3tsp
Watermelon, dark green	195	200	1 Big slice

FATS AND OILS EXCHANGE LIST

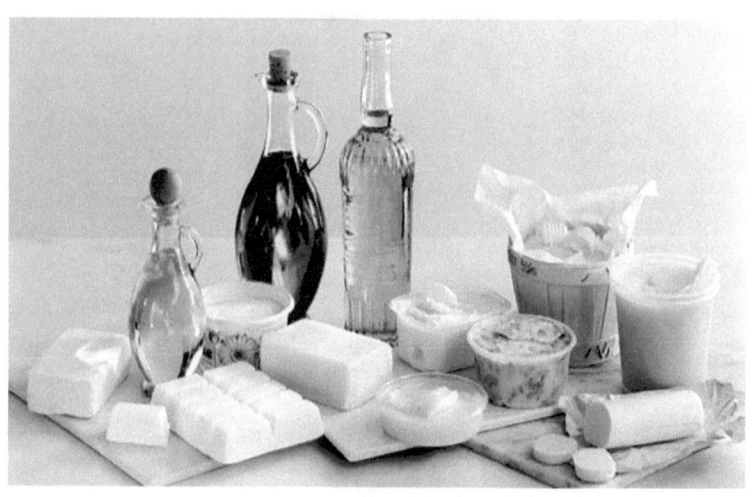

1 FATS AND OIL EXCHANGE	
Energy	72–90 kcal
Carbohydrate	Nil
Protein	Nil
Fat	8–10 g
Fiber	Nil

1 FATS AND OIL EXCHANGE LIST				
Food Ingredient	Raw weight (g)	Quantity (tsp)	Energy (kcal)	Fat (g)
Butter	10g	2tsp	72	8
Ghee(Cow)	10g	2tsp	90	10
Hydrogenated oil	10g	2tsp	90	10
Cooking Oil	10ml	2tsp	90	10

Source: NIN (1989)

SUGARS EXCHANGE LIST

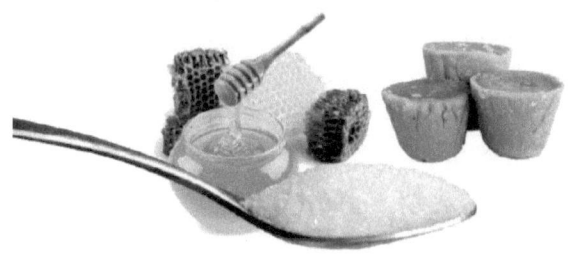

1 SUGARS EXCHANGE LIST	
Energy	16-20 kcal
Carbohydrate	4-5g
Protein	Nil
Fat	Nil
Fiber	Nil

1 SUGARS EXCHANGE LIST			
Food Ingredient	Raw weight (g)	Energy (kcal)	Carbohydrate (g)
Honey*	5	16	4
Jaggery, cane	5	18	4
Sugar*	5	20	5

Source: IFCT (2017) & NIN (1989)*

Note:

- Nutrient values have been rounded off to the nearest number
- Not Determined/Based on method of preparation
- Regional Variation on the size of fruit available (Fruit Exchange)
- Cooked Portions are approximate in quantity
- Abbreviations: tsp - Teaspoon, no - Number, kcal -Calories

References

1. Longvah, T., Ananthan, R., Bhaskarachary, K.., & Venkaiah, K. (2017). *Indian Food Composition Tables,* India, Hyderabad: National Institute of Nutrition.
2. *Gopalan, C., Sastri, B.V.R., & Balasubramanian, S. C. (1989). *Nutritive Value of Indian Foods (Rev.ed.).* India, Hyderabad: National Institute of Nutrition.

MEAL PLANNING FOOD EXCHANGE READY RECKONER

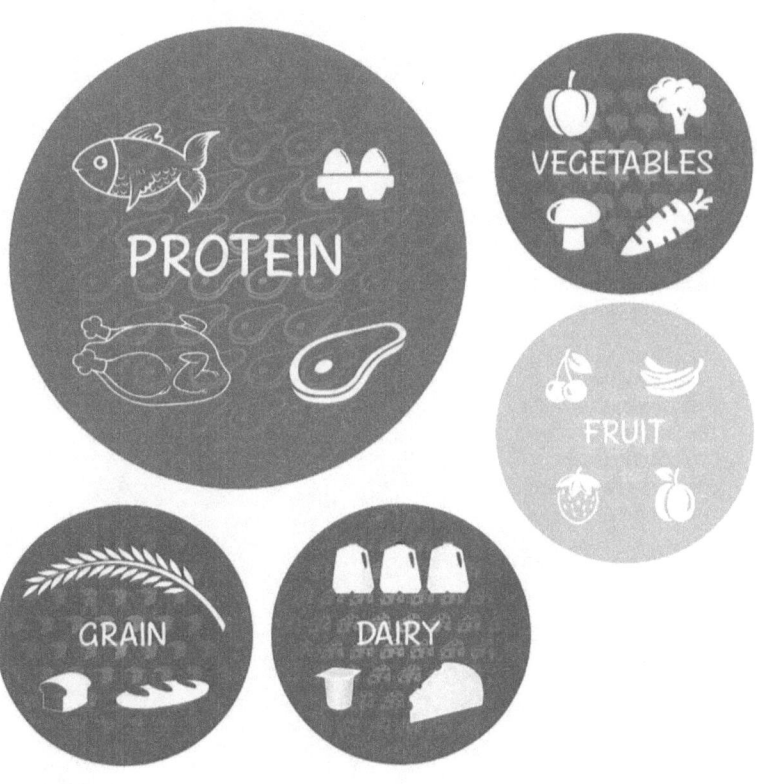

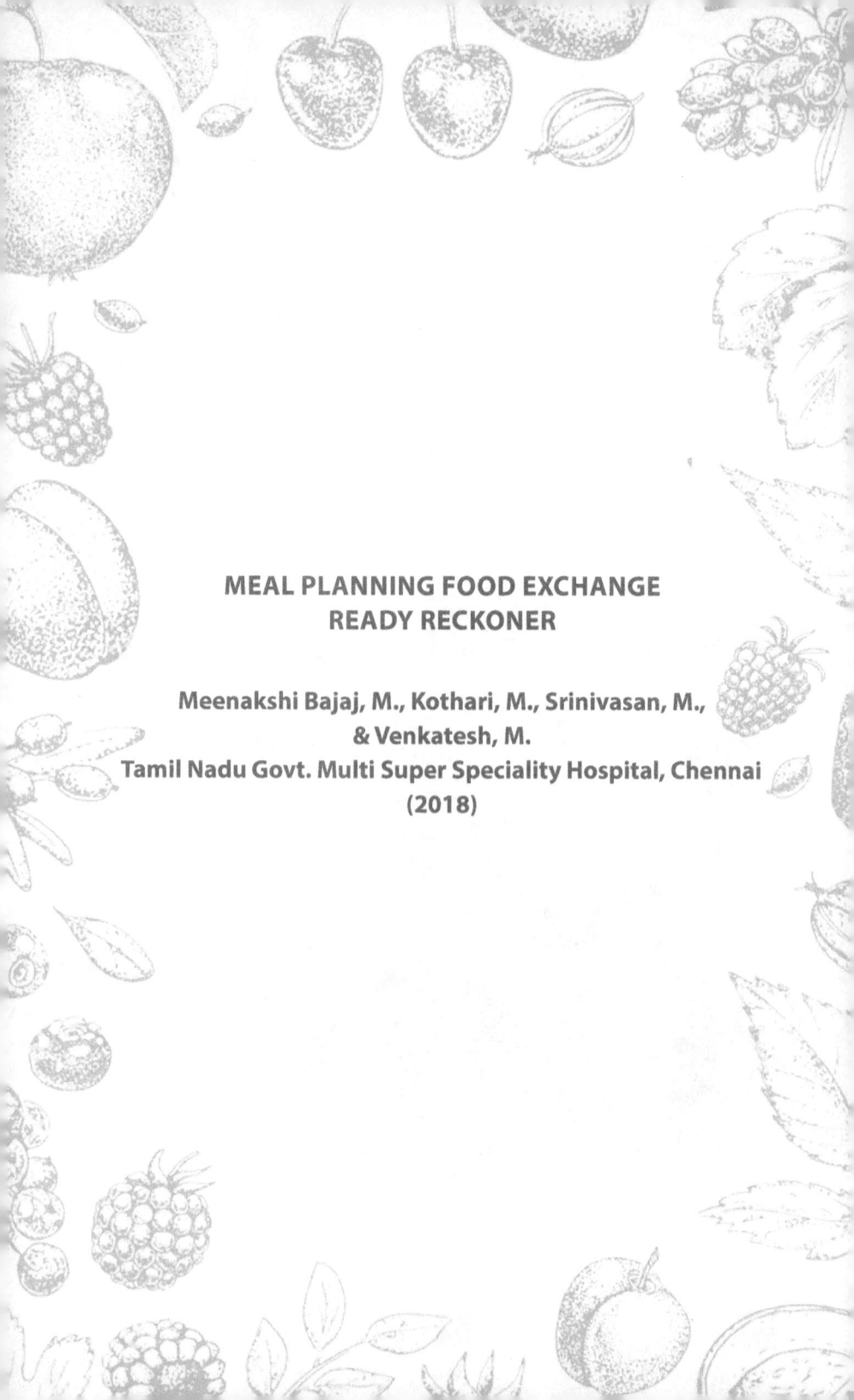

MEAL PLANNING FOOD EXCHANGE
READY RECKONER

**Meenakshi Bajaj, M., Kothari, M., Srinivasan, M.,
& Venkatesh, M.**
Tamil Nadu Govt. Multi Super Speciality Hospital, Chennai
(2018)

Food Groups (Exchange) (edible portion)	Qty (g)/ (ml)	Energy (kcal)	CHO (g)	Protein (g)	Fat (g)	Fiber (g)
Cereals & Millets	25 g	85	17	3	1	2
Pulses	25 g	80	13	6	0.5	3
Whole Grams	25 g	75	12	5	0	5
Soyabean	20 g	75	2	8	4	5
Group A (Green Leafy Vegetables)	100 g	35	3	4	1	5
Group B (Roots & Tubers)	100 g	50	10	1	0	3
Group C (Other Vegetables)	150 g	30	4	2	0	4
Fruits	90 g	40	8	1	0	3
Nuts	15 g	85	2	3	7	1
Sugars	5 g	20	5	0	0	0
Milk, Whole, Cow	100 ml	73	5	3	4	0
Skimmed Milk	100 ml	29	4	2.5	0	0
Egg, poultry, whole, raw	50 g	67	0	6.6	4.6	0
Egg, Country Hen Whole, Raw	50 g	84	0	6.6	6.5	0
Animal Meat, Marine Fish & Shellfish	75 g	75	0	13	2	0
Fat	10 g	90	0	0	10	0

Note:

- The meal planning food exchange list depicts the average value of the macronutrients of the food items in each exchange list described in the following individual exchange tables
- Nutrient values have been rounded off to the nearest number
- Abbreviation: Qty - Quantity, g - gram, ml - milliliter, Kcal - kilocalorie, CHO - Carbohydrate

References

1. Longvah, T., Ananthan, R., Bhaskarachary, K.., &Venkaiah, K. (2017). *Indian Food Composition Tables*, India, Hyderabad: National Institute of Nutrition.
2. Gopalan, C., Sastri, B.V.R., & Balasubramanian, S. C. (1989). *Nutritive Value of Indian Foods (Rev.ed.)*. India, Hyderabad: National Institute of Nutrition.

FATTY ACID CONTENT IN FOODS

FATTY ACID CONTENT IN FOODS

Meenakshi Bajaj, M., Fahmitha, N., Lavanya, B., & Mounika, G.

Tamil Nadu Govt. Multi Super Speciality Hospital, Chennai
(2018)

Dietary Fat Recommendations 1957–2015

Focus shifts from *total fat* to *type of fat*.

American Heart Association		Dietary Guidelines
1957: • 25-30% of calories from total fat. • "The possibility remains that the kind, rather than the amount of fat in the diet is responsible for atherosclerosis."	**1950**	
1961: • 25-35% of calories from total fat. • Substitute vegetable oils and PUFA for SFA. **1965:** • Eat less SFA. • Increase intake of unsaturated vegetable oils and other PUFA, substituting them for SFA wherever possible. **1968:** • Decrease SFA, increase PUFA. • <40% of calories from total fat. • "PUFA should probably comprise twice the quantity of SFA."	**1960**	
1973: • ≤35% calories from total fat. • Of that 35%, ≤10% from SFA, ≤10% from PUFA, remainder from MUFA. • "…fat calories should be distributed throughout each day…a massive high saturated fat meal is inappropriate at any time." **1978:** • 30-35% of calories from total fat. • <10% from SFA, ≤10% from PUFA, remainder from MUFA.	**1970**	
1982, 1986, 1988: • <30% of calories from total fat (1982: 30-35%). • <10% of calories from SFA. • ≤10% of calories from PUFA.	**1980**	**1980** *(inaugural edition of DGA)*, **1985:** • Avoid too much total fat and SFA.
1993: • <30% of calories from total fat. • <10% of calories from SFA • ≤10% of calories from PUFA. • Widespread consumption of very-low-fat diets not justified by current evidence. **1996:** • <30% of calories from total fat. • 8-10% of calories from SFA. • ≤10% of calories from PUFA. • ≤15% of calories from MUFA.	**1990**	**1990, 1995** • Select a diet low in total fat and SFA. • ≤30% of calories from total fat. • ≤10% calories from SFA.
2000: • ≤30% of calories from total fat. • <10% of calories from SFA. • Limit intake of TFA. • Very-low-fat (<15% of calories) diets not recommended for the general population. **2006:** • 25-35% of calories from fat is appropriate in a healthy dietary pattern. • <7% of calories from SFA. Replace with MUFA & PUFA. • <1% of calories from TFA.	**2000**	**2000:** • Choose a diet low in SFA and moderate in total fat. • ≤30% of calories from total fat. • <10% of calories from SFA. • TFA as low as possible. **2005:** • 20-35% of calories from total fat, with most fats coming from PUFA & MUFA oils. • <10% of calories from SFA. • TFA as low as possible. • Limit intake of fats & oils high in SFA & TFA, and choose products low in such fats & oils.
2013: • Advise adults who would benefit from lowering LDL cholesterol to aim for a healthy dietary pattern* that achieves 5-6% of calories from SFA. Replace with MUFA & PUFA. • Reduce % of calories from TFA.	**2010**	**2010:** • 20–35% of calories from total fat, with most coming from PUFA & MUFA. • <10% of calories from SFA. Replace them with MUFA & PUFA. • TFA as low as possible. **2015 Dietary Guidelines Advisory Committee report:** • <10% of calories from SFA. Replace with unsaturated fat, particularly PUFA. • Partially hydrogenated oils containing TFA should be avoided.

*A healthy dietary pattern emphasizes intake of vegetables, fruits, and whole grains; includes low-fat dairy products, poultry, fish, legumes, non-tropical vegetable oils, and nuts; and limits intake of sweets, sugar-sweetened beverages, and red meats.

Notes :
- *SFA = Saturated Fatty Acids, TFA = Trans Fatty Acids, MUFA = Monounsaturated Fatty Acids, PUFA = Polyunsaturated Fatty Acids*
- *Many of these recommendations include dietary cholesterol targets, but for the purposes of this paper, these are not included .*
- *References for the guidelines / recommendations in this figure are at the end of the document*

Milk & Milk Products	Raw Weight	Fat (g)	TSFA (g)	TMUFA (g)	TPUFA (g)	Cholesterol (mg)
Buffalo Milk (whole)	100 ml	7	5	2		
Buttermilk (Cow's milk) *	100 ml	1				
Cow Milk (whole)	100 ml	4	3	1		
Curd*	100 ml	4				
Paneer	100 g	15	9	4		
Skimmed milk*	100 ml					
Skimmed milk powder*	100 g					

Meat & Poultry Products	Raw Weight (g)	Fat (g)	TSFA (g)	TMUFA (g)	TPUFA (g)	Cholesterol (mg)
Beef, chops	100	7	3	3		5
Chicken, poultry, breast, skinless	100	9	1	1		6
Goat, chops	100	6	3	2		88
Egg, poultry, whole, raw	100	9	3	3	1	366

All blank spaces in the table represent below the detectable limit

CHOLESTEROL
CONTENT IN
1Eggyolk (15gms)

=

Goat chops (200gms)

Marine Products	Raw Weight (g)	Fat (g)	TSFA (g)	TMUFA (g)	TPUFA (g)	Cholesterol (mg)
Anchovy (Nethili)	100	1				30
Paarai (Jackfish)	100	2	1		1	23
Pomfret, black	100	5	2	1	1	48
Prawns, big	100	1				87
Salmon fish	100	10	4	2	2	61
Vanjaram (Seer fish)	100	5	2	1	1	68

Nuts and Oilseeds	Raw Weight (g)	Fat (g)	TSFA (g)	TMUFA (g)	TPUFA (g)	Cholesterol (mg)
Almond	100	58	4	38	13	
Cashew nut	100	45	8	28	7	
Coconut, kernel, fresh	100	41	28	2	1	
Groundnut	100	40	8	18	12	
Mustard seed	100	40	2	21	9	
Pistachio nut	100	42	4	19	12	
Walnut	100	64	5	11	45	

All blank spaces in the table represent below the detectable limit

Note:

- TSFA - Total Saturated Fatty Acid
- TMUFA - Total Mono-Unsaturated Fatty Acid
- TPUFA - Total Poly Unsaturated Fatty Acid
- Nutrient values have been rounded off to the nearest number

References

1. Longvah, T., Ananthan, R., Bhaskarachary, K.., &Venkaiah, K. (2017). *Indian Food Composition Tables*, India, Hyderabad: National Institute of Nutrition.
2. *Gopalan, C., Sastri, B.V.R., & Balasubramanian, S. C. (1989). *Nutritive Value of Indian Foods (Rev.ed.)*. India, Hyderabad: National Institute of Nutrition.

FATTY ACID CONTENT IN FOODS

Fat and Oils	Raw Weight (g)	Fat (g)	TSFA (g)	TMUFA (g)	TPUFA (g)	Cholesterol (mg)
Butter	100	81	69	28	3	

FATS AND OILS			
Oils/Fats	TSFA	TMUFA	TPUFA
Coconut Oil	89.5*	7.8	2
Corn Oil	12.7	29.6	57.4
Cotton Seed Oil	25.9	22.9	50.9
Ground Nut Oil	20.9	49.3	29.9
Mustard or Rapeseed Oil	10.7	56.0**	32.6
Olive Oil	14.8	74.5	10
Palm Oil	46.3	43.7	10
Palmolein	47.7	41.4	10.6
Rice Bran Oil	22.1	41	35.7
Safflower Oil	10.7	16.7	73.5
Gingelly Oil	13.7	41.3	44.5
Soyabean Oil	13.1	28.9	57.2
Sunflower Oil	9.1	25.1	66.2
Butter	69.4*	28	2.5
Lard	46.2*	45.2	11
Tallow	54.9*	40.9	4.2

All blank spaces in the table represent below the detectable limit

Note:

- Values are a percentage of the total methyl ester of the fatty acid
- * Includes lower chain fatty acid
- **Includes 46.5% of Erucic acid (22:1).
- TSFA - Total Saturated Fatty Acid.
- TMUFA - Total Mono-Unsaturated Fatty Acid.
- TPUFA-Total Poly Unsaturated Fatty Acid.
- Nutrient values have been rounded off to the nearest number

Reference

1. Gopalan, C., Sastri, B.V.R., & Balasubramanian, S. C. (1989). *Nutritive Value of Indian Foods (Rev.ed.)*. India, Hyderabad: National Institute of Nutrition.

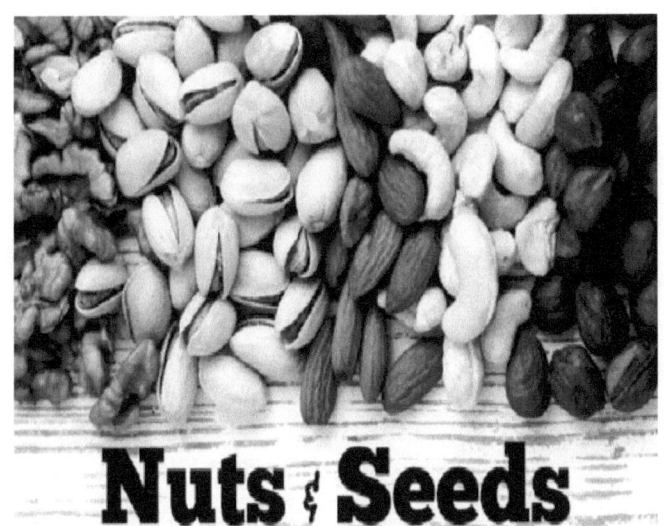

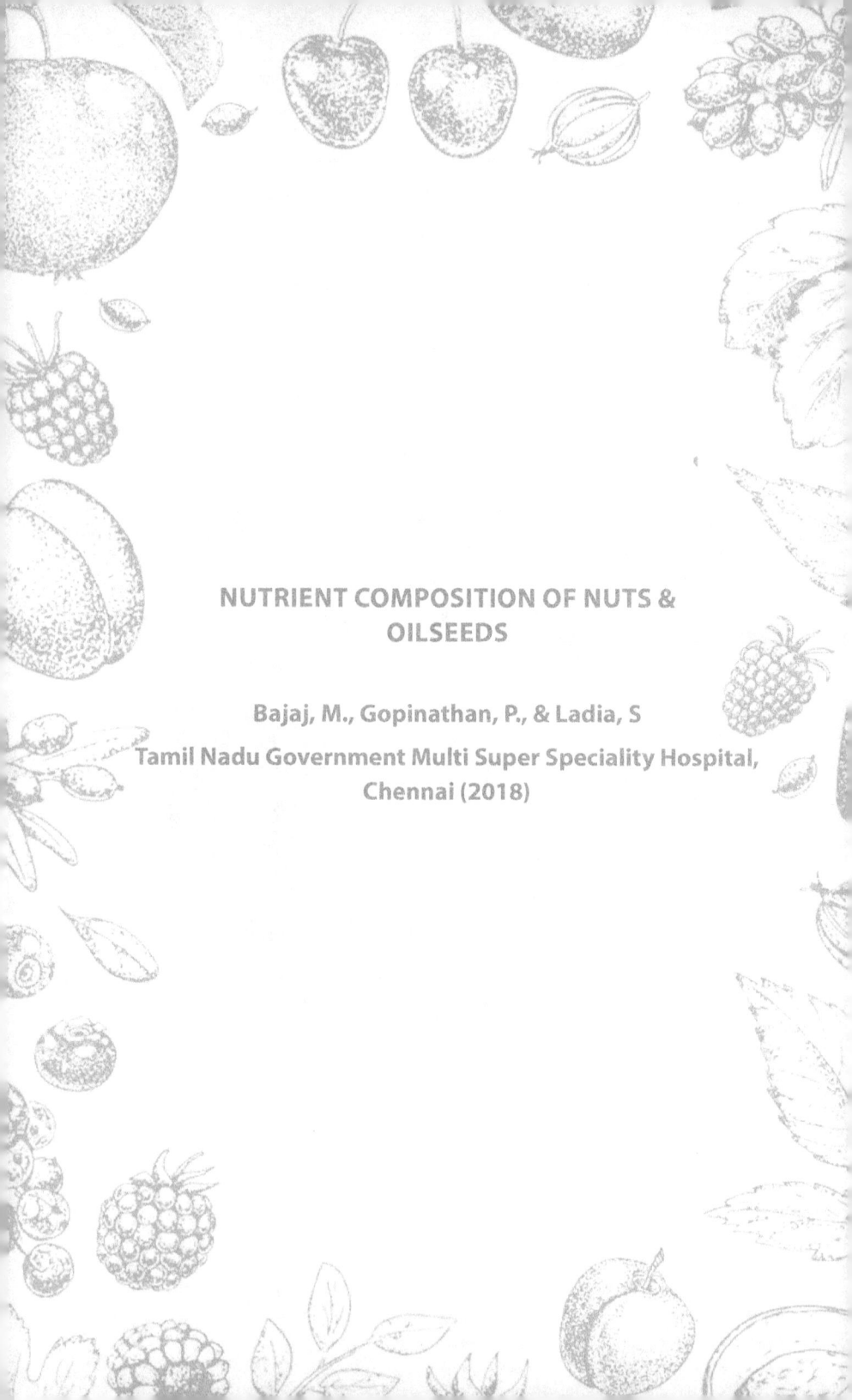

NUTRIENT COMPOSITION OF NUTS & OILSEEDS

Bajaj, M., Gopinathan, P., & Ladia, S

Tamil Nadu Government Multi Super Speciality Hospital, Chennai (2018)

NUTRITIONAL COMPOSITION / 100 g OF NUTS & OILSEEDS

	Unit	Chia Seeds	Fenugreek Seeds	Flax Seeds	Fox Nuts	Gingelly Seeds	Hemp Seeds	Melon Seeds	Pumpkin Seeds	Sunflower Seeds
Energy	kcal	490	323	534	332	573	553	557	541	584
Carbohydrate	g	44	58	29	65	23	9	15	18	20
Total Fiber	g	38	25	27	ND	12	4	ND	4	9
Insoluble Fiber	g	ND	ND	ND	ND	ND	ND	ND	ND	ND
Soluble Fiber	g	ND	ND	ND	ND	ND	ND	ND	ND	ND
Total Fat	g	31	6	42	2	50	49	47	46	52
MUFA	g	2	ND	8	0	19	5	7	14	19
PUFA	g	24	ND	29	1	22	38	28	21	23
ω 3	mg	17552	ND	ND	102	376	ND	ND	181	74
ω 6	mg	5785	ND	ND	1064	21372	ND	28092	20703	23048
SFA	g	3	2	4	0	7	5	10	9	5
Trans Fat	g	ND	ND	ND	ND	ND	ND	ND	ND	ND
Protein	g	16	23	18	15	18	32	28	25	21
Iron	mg	ND	34	6	4	15	8	7	15	5
Potassium	mg	160	770	813	1368	468	1200	648	807	645
Sodium	mg	19	67	30	5	11	5	99	18	9
Zinc	mg	4	3	4	1	8	10	10	8	5

Note:

- Nutrient values have been rounded off to the nearest number.
- 0- "Zero" The nutrient values determined are negligible.
- Abbreviation: ND – Not Determined, ω 3 – Omega 3 Fatty acid & ω 6 – Omega 6 Fatty acid

Reference

1. USDA National Nutrient Database for Standard Reference

NUTRIENT COUNTER

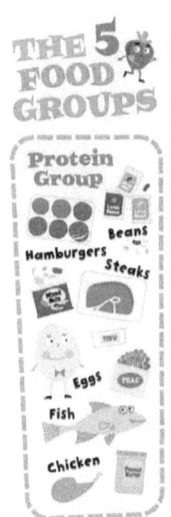

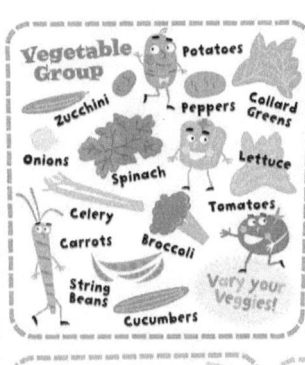

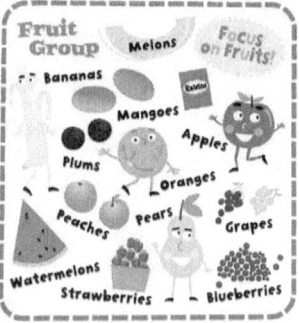

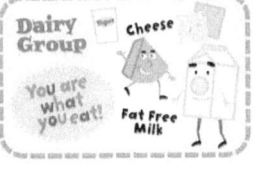

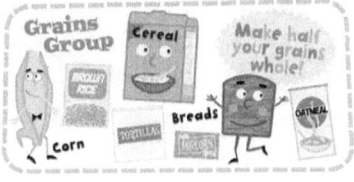

NUTRIENT COUNTER

Bajaj, M., Begam, S., & Fahmitha, N., Kothari, S., Venkatesh, M & Munusamy, V.

Tamilnadu Government Multi Super Speciality Hospital, Chennai (2018)

NUTRIENT COUNTER

$1 cup = 200\ ml$

CEREAL EXCHANGE LIST							
Food Ingredient	Quantity Raw Weight (g)	Cooked Portion+	Energy (Kcal)	CHO (g)	Protein (g)	Fat (g)	Fiber (g)
Processed cereals							
Modern sweet bread	25	1 Slice - 10cm width, Thickness- 1cm	65	13	2	1	
Kellogg's cornflakes	25	-	93	21	1		
Quaker Oats	25	-	101	17	3	2	3
Unprocessed cereals		-					
Barley	25	1 cup	79	15	3		4
Chapati, whole wheat flour	25	30g (Chapati - 1 No, medium) 6"diameter	80	16	3		3
Dosa flour (dry)	25	1 Medium	87	18	3		1
Idly flour (dry)	25	1 Large	85	18	3		2
Maize, dry	25	1/2 cup	84	16	2	1	3
Quinoa	25	1/2 cup	82	13	3	1	4
Rice flakes(dry)	25	1/3 cup	88	19	2		1
Rice, parboiled, milled	25	1/2 cup	88	19	2		1
Rice, raw, milled	25	1/2 cup	89	20	2		1
Rice, raw, brown	25	1/2 cup	88	19	2		1
Wheat, bulgur	25	-	85	17	3		2
Wheat flour, refined	25	-	88	19	3		1
Wheat, semolina (dry)	25	1/2 cup	83	17	3		2
Wheat, vermicelli (dry)	25	1/2 cup	83	18	2		2

MILLET EXCHANGE LIST

Food Ingredient	Quantity Raw Weight (g)	Cooked Portion	Energy (Kcal)	CHO (g)	Protein (g)	Fat (g)	Fiber (g)
Bajra	25	1/2 cup	87	15	3	1	3
Jowar	25	1/2 cup	78	17	2		3
Ragi	25	1/2 cup	80	17	2		3
Samai	25	1/2 cup	87	16	3	1	2
Varagu	25	1/2 cup	83	17	2	1	2

PULSE & WHOLE GRAM EXCHANGE LIST

Food Ingredient	Quantity Raw Weight (g)	Cooked Portion	Energy (Kcal)	CHO (g)	Protein (g)	Fat (g)	Fiber (g)
Bengal gram, dal	25	-	82	12	5	1	4
Bengal gram, whole	25	-	72	10	5	1	6
Black gram, dal	25	-	81	13	6		3
Black gram, whole	25	-	73	11	5		5
Cowpea, white	25	-	80	13	5		3
Green gram, dal	25	-	81	13	6		2
Green gram, whole	25	-	73	12	6		4
Horse gram, whole	25	-	82	14	5		2
Peas dry	25	-	76	12	5		4
Rajma, red	25	-	75	12	5		4
Red gram, dal	25	-	83	14	5		2
Soyabean, white	20	-	75	2	8	4	5

Source: RETRIEVED FROM IFCT (2017)

All blank spaces in the table represent below detectable limit

GROUP A-VEGETABLE EXCHANGE LIST

Food ingredient Green leafy veg.	Quantity Raw Weight (g) Per (35 kcal)	Cooked Portion	Energy (Kcal)	CHO (g)	Protein (g)	Fat (g)	Fiber (g)
Agathi leaves	50	¼ cup	35	3	4	1	4
Amaranth leaves	115	½ cup	35	3	4	1	5
Cabbage green	165	¾ cup	35	5	2	0	5
Cauliflower leaves	100	½ cup	35	3	4	0	3
Coriander leaves	110	½ cup	34	2	4	1	5
*Curry leaves	55	¼ cup	35	2	4	1	9
Drumstick leaves	50	¼ cup	34	3	3	1	4
Fenugreek leaves	100	½ cup	34	2	4	1	5
Lettuce	160	¾ cup	35	5	2		3
Mint	95	½ cup	35	2	4	1	6
Mustard leaves	115	½ cup	35	3	4	1	5
Ponnanganni	70	¾ cup	36	4	4		5
Radish leaves	135	¾ cup	35	4	3	1	2
Spinach	145	¾ cup	35	3	3	1	3

GROUP B -VEGETABLE EXCHANGE LIST

Food Ingredient Roots & Tubers	Quantity Raw Weight (g) Per (50 kcal)	Cooked Portion	Energy (Kcal)	CHO (g)	Protein (g)	Fat (g)	Fiber (g)
Beetroot	140	1/2 cup	50	9	3		5
Carrot, orange	150	1/2 cup	50	8	1	1	6
Carrot, red	130	1/2 cup	50	9	1	1	6
Colocasia	55	1/2 cup	49	10	2		2
Onion, big	100	1/2 cup	48	10	2		2
Potato, brown skin big	75	1/2 cup	52	11	1		1
Radish, round, white skin	160	1/2 cup	49	10	1		4
Sweet potato, pink, skin	50	1/2 cup	54	12	1		2
Tapioca	65	1/2 cup	52	12	1		3
Yam, elephant	60	1/2 cup	51	10	2		3

GROUP C -VEGETABLE EXCHANGE LIST

Food Ingredient Other Vegetables	Quantity Raw Weight (g) Per (28- 30kcal)	Cooked Portion	Energy (Kcal)	CHO (g)	Protein (g)	Fat (g)	Fiber (g)
Ash gourd	170	1/2 cup	30	5	1		6
Bean scarlet, tender	70	1/2 cup	30	4	2	1	3
Bitter gourd, jagged, teeth ridges, elongate	145	1/2 cup	30	4	2		5
Bottle gourd, elongate, pale green	270	1/2 cup	30	5	1		6
Brinjal-all varieties	120	1/2 cup	30	4	2		5
Broad beans	100	1/2 cup	29	2	4		9
Capsicum, green	185	1/2 cup	30	3	2	1	4
Cauliflower	130	1/2 cup	30	3	3	1	5
Cho-Cho-marrow	160	1/2 cup	30	6	1		2
Corn, Baby	40	1/2 cup	29	5	1	1	2

GROUP C -VEGETABLE EXCHANGE LIST

Food Ingredient Other Vegetables	Quantity Raw Weight (g) Per (28- 30kcal)	Cooked Portion	Energy (Kcal)	CHO (g)	Protein (g)	Fat (g)	Fiber (g)
Cucumber, green, elongate	150	1/2 cup	29	5	1		3
Drumstick	100	1/2 cup	29	4	3		7
French beans, Country	125	1/2 cup	30	3	3		5
Knol-Khol	190	1/2 cup	30	3	3	1	5
Kovai, big	170	1/2 cup	30	3	2		5
Ladies finger	110	1/4 cup	30	4	2		4
Mango, green, raw	60	1/2 cup	29	6			2
Parwar	125	1/2 cup	30	4	2		3
Plantain flower	140	1/2 cup	30	3	2	1	7
Plantain, green	35	1/2 cup	28	6			1
Plantain, stem	75	1/2 cup	30	6			2
Pumpkin, green, cylindrical	120	1/2 cup	30	5	1		3
Pumpkin, orange, round	130	1/2 cup	30	5	1		3
Ridge gourd	230	1/2 cup	30	4	2		4
Snake gourd, gourd, long, pale green	240	1/2 cup	30	3	2	1	5
Tinda, tender	220	1/2 cup	30	4	2		4
Tomato, green	145	1/2 cup	30	5	2		2
Tomato, ripe, hybrid	155	1/2 cup	30	4	1	1	3
Tomato, ripe, local	160	1/2 cup	30	5	1		3
Zucchini, green	150	1/2 cup	30	3	2	1	3

MUSHROOM EXCHANGE LIST

Food Ingredient	Quantity Raw Weight (g)	Cooked Portion	Energy (Kcal)	CHO (g)	Protein (g)	Fat (g)	Fiber (g)
Button mushroom, fresh	100	¼ cup	28	2	4		3

FRUIT EXCHANGE LIST

Food Ingredient	Quantity Raw Weight (g) Per (40 kcal)	Portion	Energy (Kcal)	CHO (g)	Protein (g)	Fat (g)	Fiber (g)
Apple, big	64	1/2 Big	40	8			2
Apricot, dried	13	-	41	9			
Banana, ripe, red	36	-	40	9			1
Avocado fruit	27	-	40	8	1	4	1
Banana, poovam	38	1/2 Medium	40	9	1		1
Cherries, red	67	-	40	8	1		1
Custard apple	41	1 Medium	41	8	1		2
Dates, processed	14	2 no	40	10			1
Fig	50	-	41	8	1		2
Gooseberry	170	-	40	7	1		13
Grapes, seeded, round, green	72	18-20 no	40	9	1		1
Grapes, seeded, round, black	66	-	40	9	1		1
Guava, pink flesh	86	-	40	8	1		6
Guava, white flesh	124	1 Medium	40	6	2		11
Jackfruit, ripe	56	3 no	40	8	2		2
Jambu fruit, ripe	72	12 no	40	9	1		2
Litchi	75	-	40	9	1		1
Muskmelon, orange flesh	173	4-5 Slices	40	7	1	1	3
Orange Pulp	108	1 Medium	40	9	1		1
Papaya, ripe	168	4 Thin long slices	40	8	1		5

FRUIT EXCHANGE LIST

Food Ingredient	Quantity Raw Weight (g) Per (40 kcal)	Portion	Energy (Kcal)	CHO (g)	Protein (g)	Fat (g)	Fiber (g)
Pear	107	1 Medium	40	9			5
Pineapple	93	1 Thick Slice	40	9			3
Plum	71	5 no	40	9			1
Sapota	55	1/2 Big	40	8	1	1	5
Strawberry	164	-	40	6	2	1	4
Sweet lime, pulp	148	-	40	8	1		3
Tamarind, pulp	14	3tsp	40	9			1
Watermelon, dark green	195	1 Big slice	40	8	1		1

MILK EXCHANGE LIST

Food Ingredient	Raw Weight (g/ml)	Quantity	Energy (Kcal)	CHO (g)	Protein (g)	Fat (g)	Fiber (g)
Buttermilk (cow's milk)*	100 ml	1/2cup	15	1	1	1	
Curd cow's milk*	100 g	1/2cup	60	3	3	4	
Milk, whole, Buffalo	100 ml	1/2cup	107	8	4	7	
Milk, whole, cow	100 ml	1/2cup	73	5	3	4	
Paneer, cow's milk	100 g	-	259	12	19	15	
Skimmed milk powder cows*	100 g	-	357	51	38		
Skimmed milk*	100 ml	1/2cup	29	4	3		

Source: *RETRIEVED FROM IFCT (2017) & NIN (1989)**

All blank spaces in the table represent below detectable limit

MEAT & POULTRY EXCHANGE LIST

Food Ingredient	Quantity Raw Weight (g)	Cooked Portion	Energy (Kcal)	CHO (g)	Protein (g)	Fat (g)	Fiber (g)
Beef, chops	65	-	95		13	4	
Chicken, poultry, breast, skinless	65	-	84		11	5	
Goat, chops	50	-	88		13	4	

EGG EXCHANGE LIST

Food Ingredient	Quantity Raw Weight (g)	Cooked Portion	Energy (Kcal)	CHO (g)	Protein (g)	Fat (g)	Fiber (g)
Egg poultry, whole, raw	50	1	67		7	5	
Egg, country hen, whole, raw	50	1	84		7	7	

MARINE EXCHANGE LIST

Food Ingredient	Quantity Raw Weight (g)	Cooked Portion	Energy (Kcal)	CHO (g)	Protein (g)	Fat (g)	Fiber (g)
Crab, sea	125	-	85	0	19	1	
Pomfret, black	69	-	85	0	13	3	
Prawns, small	120	-	85	0	16	1	
Tuna	76	-	85	0	19	1	
Mackerel	85	-	86	0	18	1	

CONDIMENTS AND SPICES EXCHANGE LIST

Food Ingredient	Quantity Raw Weight (g)	Cooked Portion	Energy (Kcal)	CHO (g)	Protein (g)	Fat (g)	Fiber (g)
Asafoetida	100	-	332	72	6	1	5
Cardamom, green	100	-	255	48	8	3	23
Chilies, green	100	-	42	6	2	1	5
Chilies, red	100	-	237	29	13	6	31

CONDIMENTS AND SPICES EXCHANGE LIST

Food Ingredient	Quantity Raw Weight (g)	Cooked Portion	Energy (Kcal)	CHO (g)	Protein (g)	Fat (g)	Fiber (g)
Cloves	100	-	187	196	6	8	35
Coriander leaves	100	-	31	2	4	1	5
Coriander seed	100	-	269	13	11	17	45
Cumin seed	100	-	304	23	14	17	30
Curry leaves	100	-	64	5	7	1	17
Fenugreek seed	100	-	235	11	25	6	48
Garlic, big clove	100	-	124	22	7	0	5
Ginger, fresh	100	-	55	9	2	1	5
Mint leaves	100	-	37	2	5	1	6
Omum	100	-	357	25	16	21	21
Pepper, black	100	-	218	36	10	3	33
Poppy seeds	100	-	423	12	20	30	27
Onion, big	100	-	48	10	2		2
Onion, small	100	-	57	12	2		1
Turmeric powder	100	-	281	49	8	5	21

FAT EXCHANGE LIST

Food Ingredient	Quantity Raw Weight (g/ml)	Cooked Portion	Energy (Kcal)	CHO (g)	Protein (g)	Fat (g)	Fiber (g)
Butter *	10g	2tsp	73			8	
Ghee, Cow *	10g	2tsp	90			10	
Oil *	10ml	2tsp	90			10	

Source: RETRIEVED FROM IFCT (2017) & NIN (1989)*

All blank spaces in the table represent below detectable limit

NUTS EXCHANGE LIST

Food Ingredient	Raw Weight (g) Per 83-85 kcal	Quantity	Energy (Kcal)	CHO (g)	Protein (g)	Fat (g)	Fiber (g)
Almond	14	12 no	85		3	8	2
Cashew nut	14.5	6 no	84	4	3	7	1
Coconut, kernel, fresh	21	4tspn	86	1	1	9	2
Groundnut	16	20 no	83	3	4	6	2
Pistachio nut	16	24 no	86	3	4	7	2
Walnut	13	5 no	87	1	2	8	1

SUGARS EXCHANGE LIST

Food Ingredient	Raw Weight (g)	Quantity	Energy (Kcal)	CHO (g)	Protein (g)	Fat (g)	Fiber (g)
Honey*	25	-	80	20			
Jaggery	25	-	88	21			
Sago*	25	-	88	22			
Sugar**	25	-	97	25			

MISCELLANEOUS EXCHANGE LIST

Food Ingredient	Volume (ml)	Quantity	Energy (Kcal)	CHO (g)	Protein (g)	Fat (g)	Fiber (g)
Coconut water	100ml	½ cup	15	3			

Source: RETRIEVED FROM IFCT (2017), NIN (1989)* & USDA (2002) **

All blank spaces in the table represent below detectable limit

Note:

- Nutrient values have been rounded off to the nearest number
- All blank spaces in the table represent below the detectable limit
- Not Determined/Based on method of preparation
- Regional Variation on the size of fruit available (Fruit Exchange)
- Abbreviations: CHO - Carbohydrate, Cm - Centimeter, g - Gram, Kcal - Kilocalorie, ml - Milliliter, No - Number, Tsp - Teaspoon, - To be determined

54

References

1. Longvah, T., Ananthan, R., Bhaskarachary, K., & Venkaiah, K. (2017). *Indian Food Composition Tables,* India, Hyderabad: National Institute of Nutrition.
2. * Gopalan, C., Sastri, B.V.R., & Balasubramanian, S. C. (1989). *Nutritive Value of Indian Foods (Rev.ed.).* India, Hyderabad: National Institute of Nutrition.
3. ** Susan, E., Gebhardt, Robin, G., & Thomas. (2002). *Nutritive Value of Foods,* U.S Department of Agriculture.

GLYCEMIC INDEX AND GLYCEMIC LOAD

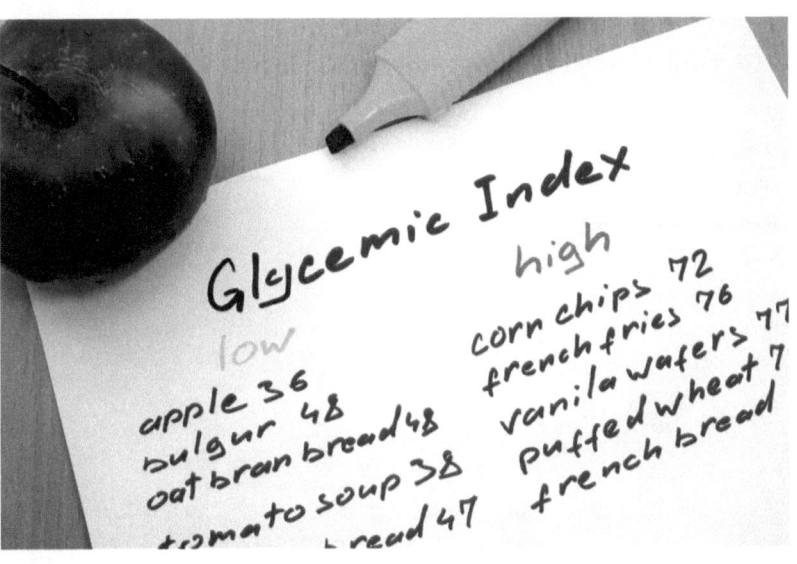

GLYCEMIC INDEX (GI)

The Glycemic Index (GI) of a food is determined by comparing its blood glucose response with the blood glucose response after a standard amount of reference food (either white bread or glucose). It is expressed as a percentage of the incremental area under the glycemic response curve elicited by a portion of food containing 50 g available carbohydrate in comparison with the area under the curve elicited by 50 g carbohydrate in the reference food of the same subject.

The GI of a food is calculated as follows:

$$\text{Glycemic Index} = \frac{\text{Incremental blood glucose area of 50 g carbohydrate test food}}{\text{Incremental blood glucose area of 50 g carbohydrate reference food}} \times 100$$

Glycemic index and glycemic load classification

	Glycemic Index (GI)	Glycemic Load (GL)
High	> 70	≥ 20
Medium	55 – 70	11 – 19
Low	< 55	≤10

Source: Atkinson. Foster-Powel., & Brand-Miller (2008); Henry &Thondre (2011)

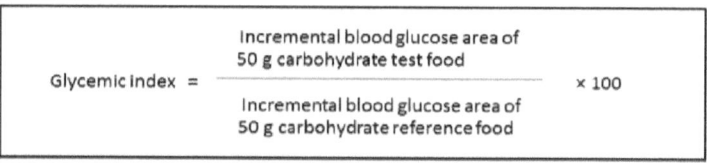

Many factors influence the GI value of foods, including the nature of the starch, the ratio of amylose to amylopectin, the degree of the retrogradation, the degree of hydration (method of cooking), particle size, food form, protein starch interaction, fat content, fiber, **antinutrients and acidity of**

foods. **Long grain basmati rice has a higher content of amylose, hence lower GI.**

In addition, other dietary factors that affect nutrient digestibility or insulin secretion, such as the fat or protein content, also influence the GI of a food.

High GI foods may increase the risk of type 2 diabetes by stimulating insulin secretion or contributing to pancreatic β- cell dysfunction, which can result in impaired glucose tolerance.

Many low GI foods are high in fiber, antioxidants and phytochemicals are beneficial to health.

Low GI diets have additionally been shown to limit reductions in insulin sensitivity. GI is not relevant to type 2 diabetes due to its direct effects on blood glucose and insulin sensitivity but also has therapeutic potential in dyslipidemia and weight management.

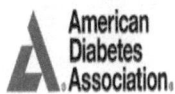

GLYCEMIC INDEX

LOW GI FOODS (55 OR LESS)

- 100% stone-ground whole wheat
- Oatmeal (rolled or steel-cut), oat bran and muesli
- Pasta converted rice, barley, and bulgar
- Sweet potato, corn, yam, lima/butter beans, peas, legumes, and lentils
- Most fruits, non-starchy vegetables and carrots

MEDIUM GI (56-69)

- Whole wheat, rye, and pita bread
- Quick Oats
- Brown and basmati rice

HIGH GI (70 OR MORE)

- White bread
- Cornflakes, puffed rice, bran flakes, and instant oatmeal
- Short grain white rice, rice pasta, macaroni and cheese from mix
- Russet potato and pumpkin
- Rice cakes and popcorn
- Melons

It is important to note that all foods low in GI need not necessarily be healthy, to understand this concept better a fried snack has lower GI compared to a steamed food, whole wheat puri/ paratha is lower GI than whole wheat flour phulka.

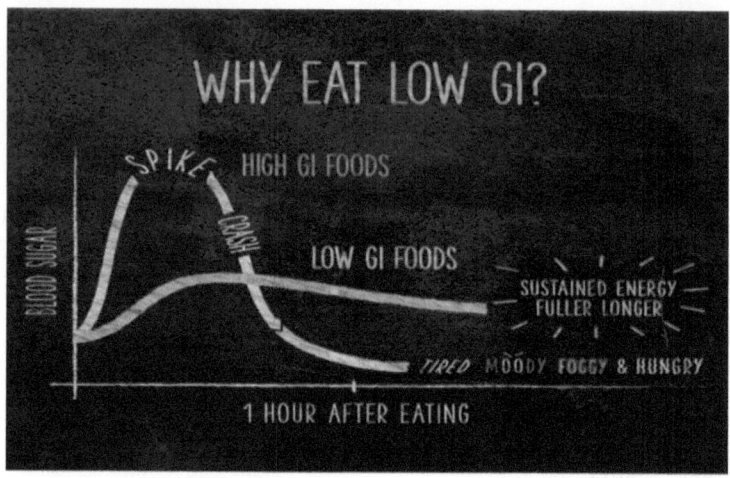

Consumption of low GI foods may be effective in the prevention and management of type 2 diabetes and may have a role in reducing the comorbidities associated with diabetes, such as cardiovascular diseases and obesity.

References

1. Goff, L., Dyson, P., & Whelan, K. (Eds.). (2016).*Advanced Nutrition and Dietetics in Diabetes*, (1ᵗed.). John Wiley & Sons, Ltd, UK: West Sussex.
2. Henry, C.J.K &Thondre, P.S. (2011). The glycaemic index: concept, recent developments and its impact on diabetes and obesity. In Pasternak, C.A. (Ed), St. Ives, Cambridge shire: Smith – Gourdon.
3. Atkinson, F.S., Foster- Powell, K., & Brand-Miller., J.C.(2008). International table of glycemic index and glycemic load values, *Diabetes Care, 31*, 2281-2283.

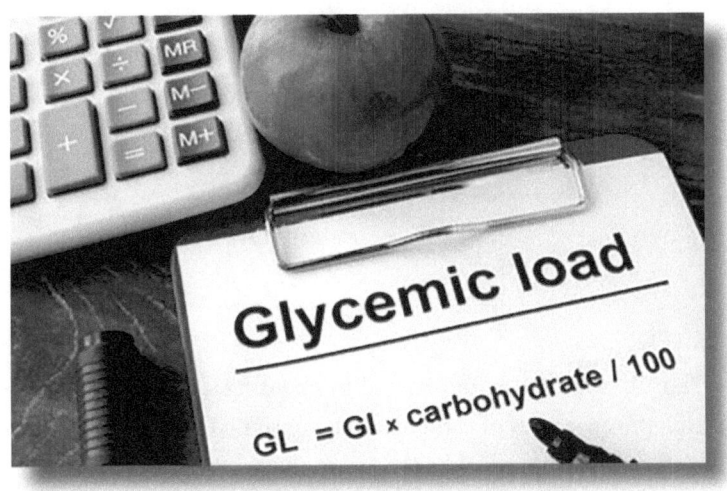

GLYCEMIC LOAD (GL)

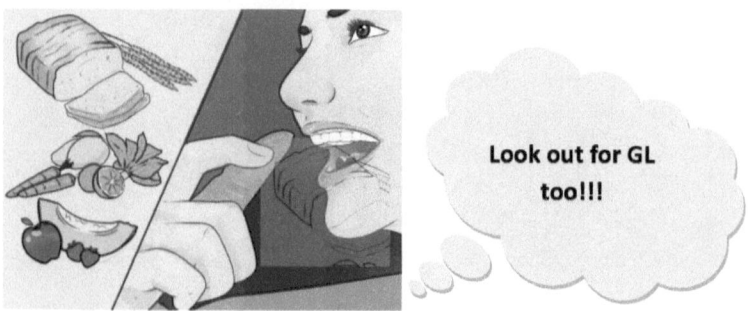

The concept of glycemic load (GL) was first introduced by researchers at Harvard University to quantify the glycemic impact of a portion of food.

Glycemic load is based on the glycemic index (GI) and is calculated by multiplying the grams of available carbohydrate in the food to the food's GI and then dividing by 100.

$$\text{Glycemic Load} = \frac{\text{GI} \times \text{amount of CHO in the portion consumed in the meal}}{100}$$

The GL of a diet can be lowered by choosing foods with low GI or by reducing the quantities of carbohydrates consumed or by a combination of both. For example, rice cooked in a pressure cooker is of a higher glycemic load than rice cooked by straining method due to maximum retention of carbohydrates.

Though Apple has a lower GI (36) and lowers GL (5) when compared to pineapple lower GI (59) and lower GL (9), one needs to ensure not to increase the quantity of apple as this may further raise the GL. Hence the concept of consuming low GI, low GL food will be lost if the portion size is not retained.

Glycemic Load (GL)

No negative effects have been demonstrated so far by following a low GI with healthy ingredients or low GL diet with healthy ingredients.

The GL of a typical serving of food is the product of the amount of available carbohydrate in that serving and the GI of the food. The higher the GL, the greater the expected elevation in blood glucose and in the insulinogenic effect of the food. The long-term consumption of a diet with a relatively high GL (adjusted for total energy) is associated with an increased risk of type 2 diabetes and coronary heart disease.

Reference

1. Goff, L., Dyson, P., & Whelan, K. (Eds.). (2016). *Advanced Nutrition and Dietetics in Diabetes*, (1ˢᵗed.). John Wiley &Sons, Ltd, UK: West Sussex.

GLYCEMIC INDEX AND GLYCEMIC LOAD

Bajaj, M., Kothari, S., & Vijayalakshmi, M.

Tamil Nadu Government Multi Super Specialty Hospital, Chennai (2018)

Sugars	Glycemic Index (Glucose = 100)	Serving Size (g)	Available Carbohydrate (g/serve)	Glycemic Load (GL/Serve)
Fructose (50g)	20	10	10	2
Dextrose (50g) **	85	10	10	9
Sucrose (25g) *	110	10	10	11

Fruits	Glycemic Index (Glucose = 100)	Serving Size (g)	Available Carbohydrate (g/serve)	Glycemic Load (GL/serve)
Apple (mean of 5 studies)	36	120	14	5
Apricots, dried	32	60	30	10
Banana (mean of 9 studies)	48	120	24	11
Cherries, raw, sour	22	120	12	3
Dates, (Khalas variety),dried processed vacuum packed, U.A.E(mean of 5 studies)	36	60	45	16
Kiwifruit *	47	120	12	6
Mango, ripe ***	60	120	15	9
Orange (mean of 5 studies)	45	120	11	5
Papaya, ripe ***	60	120	29	17
Pear (mean of 4 studies)	38	120	11	4
Pineapple *	51	120	16	8
Raisins	66	60	43	28

Raw Food Ingredients	Glycemic Index (Glucose =100)	Serving Size (g)	Available Carbohydrate (g/serve)	Glycemic Load (GL/serve)
Bajra	49	75	50	25
Barley	48	150	42	20
Kidney Beans	19	150	25	5
Maize	59	30	13	8
Pea Green	54	80	7	4
Rajmah	19	150	30	6

Cooked Foods	Glycemic Index (Glucose =100)	Serving Size (g)	Available Carbohydrate (g/serve)	Glycemic Load (GL/serve)
Bajra (Roti)	67	NA	NA	NA
Bengal Gram, Dhal(Chick Pea)	11	150	36	4
Chapati, (thin, wheat flour), with green gram dhal	81	200	50	41
Chapati, (wheat) served with bottle ground and tomato curry	66	60	32	21
Chapati, maize	64	64	NA	NA
Chappati, Bajra	49	NA	NA	NA
Chappati, Barley	49	NA	NA	NA
Chappati, Maize	59	NA	NA	NA
Cheela Bengal Gram	42	150	28	12
Cheela Green Gram	45	150	26	12
Dosai (parboiled and raw rice + black dhal, soaked, ground, fermented, pan fried) with chutney	77	250	52	40
Dosai (parboiled and raw rice, soaked, ground, fermented & steamed) with chutney	77	150	39	30
Idly (parboiled, raw rice, black dhal, soaked, grounded, fermented with chutney)	60	250	52	31
Jowar Roti	77	NA	NA	NA
Pongal (Rice and roasted green gram dhal, pressure cooked)	90	250	52	47
Poori with potato masala	82	150	41	34
Potato (Steamed)	65	150	27	18
Puttu with Bengal gram curry	79	250	74	58
Rice (Boiled) White	43	150	38	16
Tapioca (Steamed)	70	250	18	12
Upma	67	150	42	28
Varagu, pressure cooked	68	76	50	34
Whole Wheat Kernel	30	50	38	11

GL is estimated by multiplying the food's listed GI value with glucose as the reference food by the listed g carbohydrate per serving and dividing by 100.

Note:

- *Portions of the test food and the reference food contained 25 g carbohydrate.
- ** GI calculated from the 180 min AUC data included in the original article using the AUC food/AUC reference food formula.
- *** Portions of the test food and the reference food contained 75 g carbohydrate.

- NA - Not available

Reference

1. Atkinsons, F.S., Fostein NA Powell, K.,& Miller, B. J.C. (2008). International Tables of Glycemic Index and Glycemic Load values, *Diabetes Care, 31*(12).

GLYCEMIC INDEX AND GLYCEMIC LOAD OF INDIAN FOODS

Bajaj, M., & Gopinathan, P .

Tamil Nadu Government Multi Super Specialty Hospital, Chennai (2018)

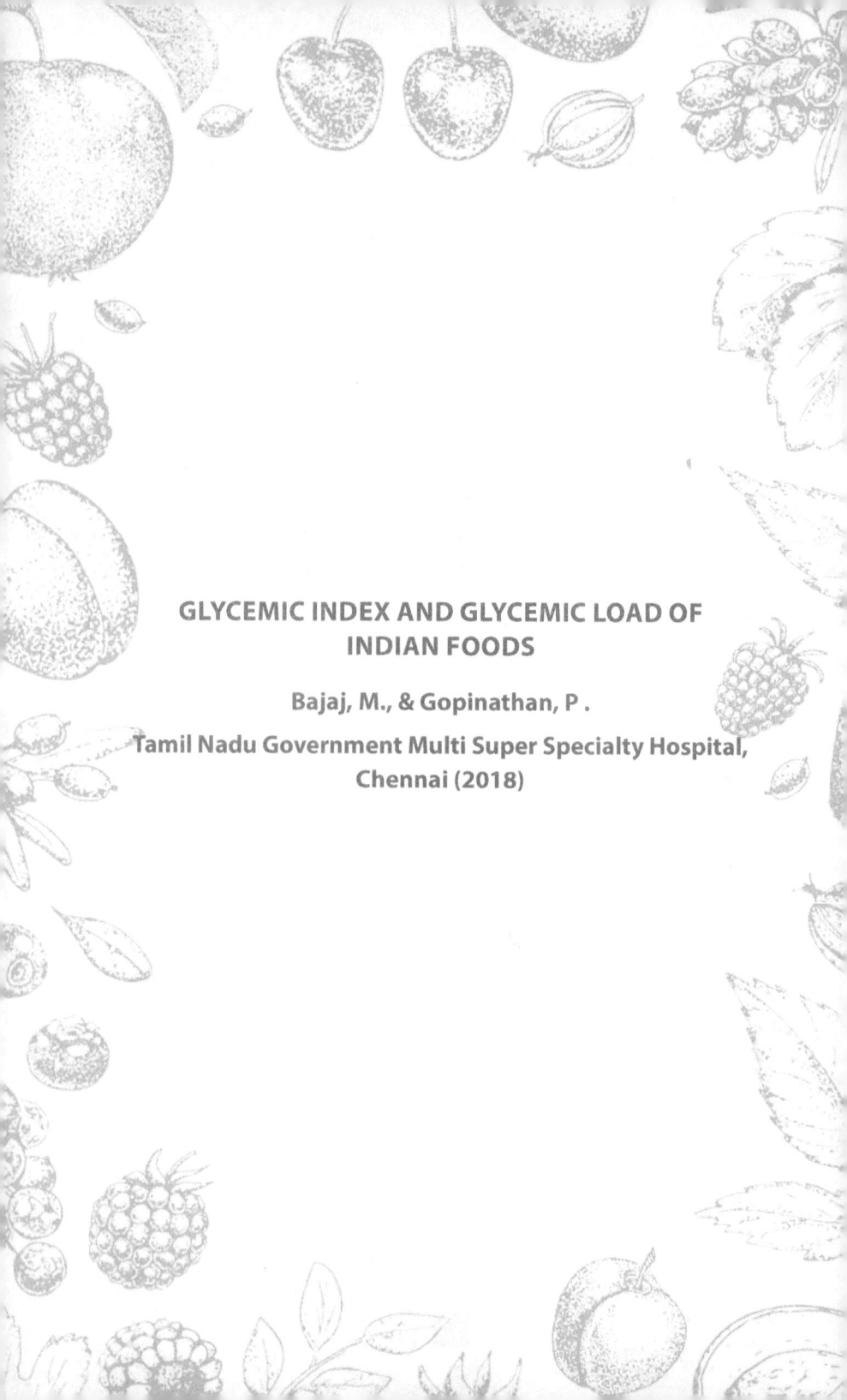

FOOD INGREDIENTS WITH LOW GLYCEMIC LOAD (<10)

Food Ingredients	CHO/100g	Glycemic Index	Glycemic Load
Apple, big	13	36	5
Beetroot	6	64	4
Broccoli, raw	7	10	1
Cabbage, green	3	10	0
Capsicum, green	2	10	0
Carrot, orange	6	16	1
Cashew nut	25	25	6
Cauliflower	2	6	0
Coconut, Kernel, fresh	6	45	3
Flaxseed	11	36	4
Grapes, seeded, round, black	13	59	8
Grapes, seeded, round, green	12	43	5
Kiwi	15	52	8
Lettuce	3	7	0
Maize, tender, sweet	16	52	8
Mango, green, raw	11	51	6
Onion, small	12	10	1
Orange, pulp	8	43	3
Papaya, ripe	5	60	3
Peach	8	28	2
Pineapple	9	59	5
Plum	12	69	8
Pumpkin, Orange, Round	4	75	3
Soya bean, Brown	13	16	2
Spinach	2	12	0
Strawberry	3	40	1
Tomato, ripe	3	15	0
Watermelon, pale green	3	76	2

FOOD INGREDIENTS WITH LOW GLYCEMIC LOAD (<10)

Food Ingredients	CHO/100g	Glycemic Index	Glycemic Load
Groundnut, roasted	17	14	2
Milk, buffalo's	8	39	3
Mushrooms	4	10	0
Skimmed milk, liquid	4	37	1
Walnut	10	15	2

FOOD INGREDIENTS WITH MEDIUM GLYCEMIC LOAD (10–19)

Food Ingredients	CHO/100g	Glycemic Index	Glycemic Load
Barley	61	28	17
Lentil Dhal	53	32	17
Sweet potato, pink skin	24	48	12

FOOD INGREDIENTS WITH HIGH GLYCEMIC LOAD (≥20)

Food Ingredients	CHO/100g	Glycemic Index	Glycemic Load
Dates, processed	68	103	70
Glucose syrup	78	103	80
Honey	79	61	48
Rice, parboiled, milled	77	73	56
Rice, raw, brown	78	72	56
Sago	87	70	61
Wheat bread, brown	49	74	36
Wheat bread, white	52	75	39

Source: IFCT(2017), *NTUITIVE,NIN 2018

Note

- Glycemic Load is calculated based on the information on GI of the food ingredient & Carbohydrate content in the food ingredient
- Abbreviation: CHO Carbohydrate, g gram

"GLUTEN FREE, GLYCEMIC & CARDIAC FRIENDLY HEALTHY SNACKING OPTION

"Calcium & Protein rich, Moderate in Fiber & Glycemic Load & Low in Sodium."

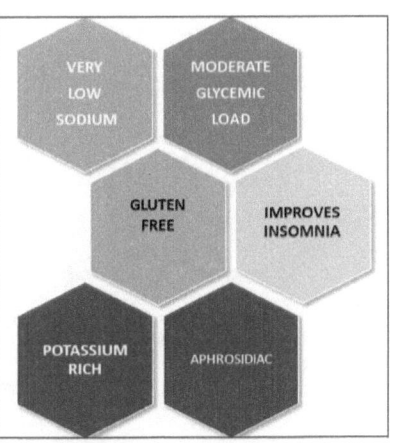

Makhana (Euryale ferox) is an aquatic crop known commonly as Gorgon Nut or Fox Nut Makhana seeds can be consumed in raw, roasted or ground form. The puffed seeds alternate dry roasted snacks. They can be soaked in water overnight, pureed and added as thickener for soups, orgravies. It can also be ground and added to soybean, bajra and jowar flours to prepare gluten free, protein rich roti.

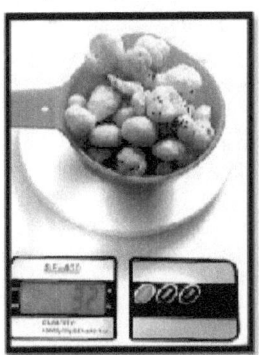

Serving size: 1 Cup (32g)	
Nutrients	**Qty**
Energy	106 Kcal
Carbohydrate	20.6 g
Total Fat	0.6 g
Protein	4.9 g
Calcium	52.2 mg
Magnesium	67.2 mg
Phosphorus	200 mg
Sodium	1.6 mg
Potassium	438 mg

References

1. Longvah, T., Ananthan, R., Bhaskarachary, K., & Venkaiah, K. (2017). *Indian Food Composition Tables*, India, Hyderabad: National Institute of Nutrition.

2. *(NTUITIVE) Nutrify India (2018), India, Hyderabad: National Institute of Nutrition.

3. International Journal of Ayurveda and Pharmaceutical Chemistry 2016

CARBOHYDRATE COUNTING

What is carb counting ?

Estimate carb content
of the food

Adjust the insulin dose
to match the amount of carbs

**Carbohydrate counting can help you choose what and
how much to eat**

CARBOHYDRATE COUNTING

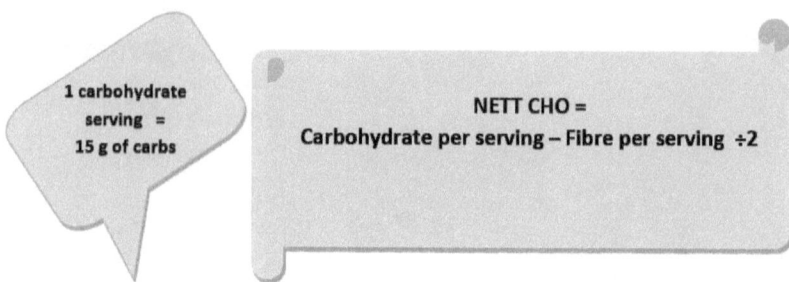

1 carbohydrate serving = 15 g of carbs

NETT CHO =
Carbohydrate per serving – Fibre per serving ÷2

Carbohydrate counting is a meal planning approach used to manage diabetes. (Edwards, 2015). Carbohydrate counting is also called 'carb counting'.

Foods that contain carbohydrates have the greatest effect on the blood glucose compared to foods that contain protein or fat. Hence there is a need to focus on the total amount of carbohydrates that can be consumed on a day in the form of meals and snacks.

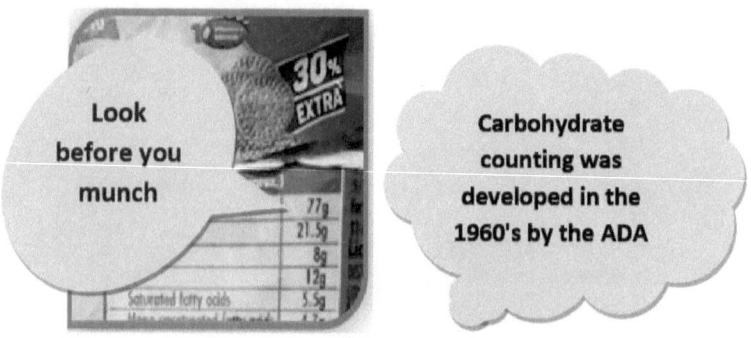

Look before you munch

Carbohydrate counting was developed in the 1960's by the ADA

1 carbohydrate count = 15 grams of carbs (approx.)

Serving sizes can be checked with measuring cups, spoons, a food scale or by using the Food exchange list or Nutrition Facts label on a food package.

Carbohydrate counting enables individuals to assess the impact of different meals on blood glucose levels and their resultant bolus insulin requirements. Carbohydrate counting can be used by anyone with diabetes, not only restricted to insulin-dependent diabetics.

Randomized control trials have shown that carbohydrate counting can improve glycemic control and quality of life without increasing the risk of hyperglycemia, weight gain or dyslipidemia. (Edwards, 2015; Tascini, Berioli, Cerquiglini, Santi, Mancini, Rogari, Toni, & Esposito, 2008).

References

1. Edwards, A.(2015). An introduction to carbohydrate counting in type 1 diabetes, *Journal of Diabetes Nursing, 19*, 73–7.
2. Tascini, G., Berioli, M.G., Cerquiglini, L., Santi, E., Mancini, G., Rogari, F., Toni, G., &Esposito, S.(2008). Carbohydrate Counting in Children and Adolescents with Type 1 Diabetes. *Nutrients, 10*, 109.

Counting carbohydrates with an insulin-to-carbohydrate ratio is valuable for tight glycemic control!

INSULIN CARBOHYDRATE RATIO (ICR)

ICR allows to easily figure out how much of short or fast-acting insulin is needed for the amount of carbohydrate one consumes. One may adjust the ratio by finding the blood glucose before and after the meal and counting the carbohydrates (CHO) taken at a meal or one may also use the Rule 500. [1]

RULE 500: CARBOHYDRATE COUNT

Assuming an average person consumes 500g carbs/ day approximately.

Example 1: If you take a total of 25 units of insulin in a typical day, each unit of insulin would cover approximately 20 grams of carbohydrate ICR= 1:20(500/ 25 = 20).

1 Cho Count = 20

Example 2: If you take 60 units daily, your ICR would be 1 unit per 8 grams of carbs 1:8

(500 / 60 = 8).

1 Cho Count =8

Rule of 500

CHO Count   =   no. of grams of carbohydrate handled by 1 unit of insulin.

CHO Count   =   500/TDD

TDD   =   Total Daily Dose of Insulin

500   =   Constant value

Your insulin-to-carb ratio can change with changes in your body weight and activity levels.

Now you can calculate Insulin requirement per meal. For Example

$$\text{Insulin requirement per meal (A)} = \frac{\text{Total g of Carbohydrate to be consumed (90g)}}{\text{Insulin to Carb Ratio (15)}} = 6U$$

INSULIN SENSITIVITY FACTOR (ISF)

ISF is used to calculate the amount of insulin you need to bring your blood glucose into the target range. This adjusts or corrects a blood glucose level that may be higher or lower than desired before a meal.[2] This can be calculated with the Rule 1800 when the blood glucose is measured as mg/dl (or Rule 100 for mmol/L).

Rule of 1800

$$ISF = \frac{1800}{\text{Total Daily Dose of Insulin}}$$

For example; 1800/60 units of Insulin gives an Insulin Sensitivity Factor of 30mg/ dl which means 1 Unit of Insulin reduces the blood glucose by 30mg/ dl. [3]

The use of Rule depends on the type of Insulin used by the patient:

Rule 1800 is used for Insulin Analogues

Rule 1500 is used for other types of Insulin

Insulin sensitivity factor can be calculated only for people with Type 1 diabetes. It cannot be calculated reliably for people with Type 2 diabetes, whose pancreas often still make some insulin and who have varying degrees of insulin resistance.

Using ISF, you can now calculate the correction dose to determine the total requirement of insulin by the patient. This correction dose is added to, or subtracted from, the pre-meal insulin dose.

Insulin Correction dose per meal (B): For example;

$$\text{Correction dose} = \frac{\text{Current Blood Glucose}(170) - \text{Target Blood Glucose}(140)}{\text{Insulin Sensitivity Factor }(30)}$$
$$= \text{Additional 1U of Pre-meal Insulin}$$

Adding the insulin dose for food (A = 6U) with the correction dose (B= 1U) gives you the total amount of insulin required by your body for that meal to maintain the target glucose levels.

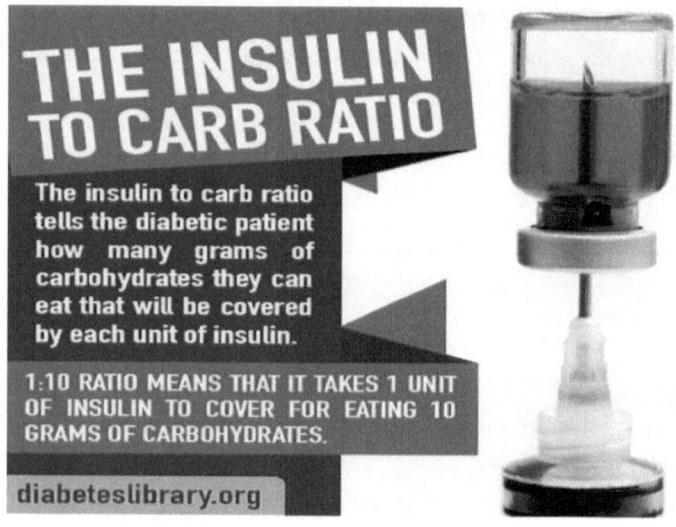

References

1. Gary Scheiner MS. Nov 2007. CDE – Integrated Diabetes Services LLC. *Insulin to Carb Ratios made Easy.* Page 1 – 3.

2. Academy of Nutrition & Dietetics. 2015. Diabetes Care & Education – *A nutrition resource for living well with diabetes.* Handout.

3. Journal of Diabetes Science & Technology, Mar 2017. RagnarHanas and Peter Adolfsson. *Bolus Calculator Settings in Well-Controlled Prepubertal Children Using Insulin Pumps Are Characterized by Low Insulin to Carbohydrate Ratios and Short Duration of Insulin Action Time,* 11(2): 247–252.

CARBOHYDRATE COUNTING

Bajaj, M., Kothari, S., & Sherene, G.

Tamil Nadu Government Multi Super Speciality Hospital, Chennai (2018).

CARBOHYDRATE COUNTING

CHO Count	CHO (g)
Free food (don't count)	0–5
½	6–10
1	11–20
1 ½	21–25
2	26–35
2 ½	36–44
3	45
3 ½	46–59
4	60
4 ½	61–74
5	75
5 ½	76–89
6	90
6 ½	91–104
7	105

Note:

- Nutrient values have been rounded off to the nearest number
- Carbohydrate count as per Food Exchange List

References

1. Carbohydrate Counting for Traditional South Asian Foods. (n.d.). Retrieved from http://www.sjsu.edu/people/ashwini.wagle/Southasians/Carbohydrate%20 Counting%20Tool%20for%20South%20Asians%204th%20Version.pdf

2. Gopalan, C., Sastri, B.V.R., & Balasubramanian, S.C. (1989). *Nutritive Value of Indian Foods (Rev.ed.)*. India, Hyderabad: National Institute of Nutrition.

3. Holzmeister, L.A. (2010). The diabetes carbohydrate and fat gram guide. *Academy of Nutrition and Dietetics (AND)*.

4. Warsaw, H.S. &Kulkarni, K. (2011). ADA complete guide to carbohydrate counting. Retrieved from http://www.diabetes.org/food-and-fitness/food/what-can-ieat/ understanding-carbohydrates/carbohydrate-counting.html

CARBOHYDRATE COUNTING
OF DIFFERENT FOOD GROUPS

CEREALS						
Cereals	Raw Weight (g)	Cooked Portion	CHO (g)	Fiber (g)	NETT CHO (g)	CHO Count
Barley	25	1 Cup	15	4	17	1
Bread, Modern	25	1 Slice- 10cm width; Thickness- 1cm	12	0	12	1
Chapati, Whole Wheat Flour	25	1 Medium	16	3	18	1
Cornflakes, Kellogg's	25	1/2 cup	21	0	21	1 ½
Dosa Flour (Dry)	25	1 Medium	18	2	19	1
Idly Flour (Dry)	25	1 Large	18	2	19	1
Oats, Quaker	25	1/3 cup	17	3	19	1
Quinoa	25	1/3 cup	13	4	15	1
Rice, Basmati (India Gate)	25	1/2 cup	19	0	19	1
Rice, Basmati (Kohinoor)	25	1/2 cup	19	1	20	1
Rice Flakes (Dry)	25	1/3 cup	19	1	20	1
Rice, Parboiled Milled	25	1/2 cup	19	1	20	1
Rice, Raw Milled	25	1/2 cup	20	1	21	1 ½
Roasted Vermicelli (Dry)	25	-	19	2	20	1
Wheat Flour (Aashirvaad)	25	-	19	3	21	1 ½
Wheat Flour (Pillsbury)	25	-	18	3	20	1
Wheat Flour, Refined	25	-	19	1	20	1
Wheat, Semolina (Dry)	25	1/2 cup	17	2	18	1
Wheat, Vermicelli (Dry)	25	1/2 cup	18	2	19	1

MILLETS

Cereals	Raw Weight (g)	Cooked Portion	CHO (g)	Fiber (g)	NETT CHO (g)	CHO Count
Bajra	25	1/2 Cup	15	3	17	1
Jowar	25	1/2 Cup	17	3	19	1
Ragi	25	1/2 Cup	17	3	19	1
Samai	25	1/2 Cup	16	2	17	1
Varagu	25	1/2 Cup	17	2	18	1

PULSES

Pulses	Raw Weight (G)	CHO (g)	Fiber (g)	NETT CHO (g)	CHO Count
Bengal gram, dhal	25	12	4	14	1
Bengal gram, whole	25	10	6	13	½
Black gram, dhal	25	13	3	15	1
Black gram, whole	25	11	5	14	½
Cowpea, white	25	13	3	15	1
Green gram, dhal	25	13	2	14	1
Green gram, whole	25	12	4	14	1
Horse gram, whole	25	14	2	15	1
Peas dry	25	12	4	14	1
Rajmah, red	25	12	4	14	16
Red gram, dhal	25	14	2	15	1
Soyabean, white	22.5	2	5	5	0

VEGETABLES – GREEN LEAFY VEGETABLES

Group A (Green Leafy Vegetables)	Raw Weight (g) / 35kcal	Cooked Portion	CHO (g)	Fiber (g)	NETT CHO (g)	CHO Count
Agathi leaves	50	1/4 cup	3	5	6	½
Amaranth leaves, green	100	1/2 cup	2	4	4	0
Cabbage, green	150	3/4 cup	6	3	8	½
Cauliflower leaves	100	1/2 cup	4	4	6	½
Drumstick leaves	50	1/4 cup	3	4	5	0
Fenugreek leaves	100	1/2 cup	2	5	5	0
Gogu Leaves, Red	95	1/2 cup	4	1	5	0
Lettuce	150	3/4 cup	5	3	7	½
Mustard leaves	100	1/2 cup	2	4	4	0
Parsley	45	1/4 cup	4	1	5	0
Ponnanganni	70	1/3 cup	4	5	7	½
Radish leaves	125	2/3 cup	3	3	5	0
Spinach	125	2/3 cup	3	3	5	0

VEGETABLES – ROOTS AND TUBERS

Group B (Roots and Tubers)	Raw Weight (g) / 50-55 kcal	Cooked Portion	CHO (g)	Fiber (g)	NETT CHO (g)	CHO Count
Beetroot	140	½ cup	9	5	12	1
Carrot, orange	150	½ cup	8	6	11	1
Carrot, red	130	½ cup	9	6	12	1
Colocasia	60	½ cup	11	2	12	1
Potato, brown skin big	75	½ cup	11	1	12	1
Sweet potato, pink skin	50	½ cup	12	2	13	´1
Radish, round, white skin	160	½ cup	10	4	12	1
Tapioca	65	½ cup	12	3	14	1
Yam, elephant	60	½ cup	10	3	12	1

VEGETABLES – OTHER VEGETABLES

Group C (Other Vegetables)	Raw Weight (g) / 25–30 kcal	Cooked Portion	CHO (g)	Fiber (g)	NETT CHO (g)	CHO Count
Ash gourd	170	1/2 cup	5	6	8	½
Beans scarlet, tender	70	1/2 cup	4	3	6	½
Bitter gourd, jagged, teeth ridges, elongate	145	1/2 cup	4	5	7	½
Bottle gourd, elongate, pale green	270	1/2 cup	5	6	8	½
Brinjal all varieties	110	1/2 cup	4	4	6	½
Broad beans	100	1/2 cup	2	9	7	½
Capsicum, green	175	1/2 cup	3	4	5	0
Cauliflower	130	1/2 cup	3	5	6	½
Cho- Cho- marrow	150	1/2 cup	5	2	6	½
Corn, Baby	40	1/2 cup	5	2	6	½
Cucumber, green, elongate	150	1/2 cup	5	3	7	½
Drumstick	100	1/2 cup	4	7	8	½
French beans, Country	120	1/2 cup	3	5	6	½
Knol-Khol	175	1/2 cup	2	5	5	0
Koval, big	170	1/2 cup	3	5	6	½
Ladies finger	110	1/4 cup	4	4	6	½
Mango, green, raw	60	1/2 cup	6	2	7	½
Onion, stalk	100	1/2 cup	3	5	6	½
Parwar	125	1/2 cup	4	3	6	½
Plantain flower	140	1/2 cup	3	7	7	½

VEGETABLES – OTHER VEGETABLES

Group C (Other Vegetables)	Raw Weight (g) / 25–30 kcal	Cooked Portion	CHO (g)	Fiber (g)	NETT CHO (g)	CHO Count
Plantain, green	35	1/2 cup	6	1	7	½
Plantain, stem	75	1/2 cup	6	2	7	½
Pumpkin, green, cylindrical	121	1/2 cup	5	3	7	½
Pumpkin, orange, round	125	1/2 cup	5	3	7	½
Ridge gourd	230	1/2 cup	4	4	6	½
Snake gourd, long, pale green	240	1/2 cup	3	5	6	½
Tinda, tender	200	1/2 cup	4	4	6	½
Tomato, green	145	1/2 cup	5	2	6	½
Tomato, ripe, hybrid	150	1/2 cup	5	2	6	½
Tomato, ripe, local	150	1/2 cup	4	3	6	½
Zucchini, green	150	1/2 cup	3	3	5	0

FRUITS

Fruits	Raw Weight (g) / 40 kcal	Portion Size	CHO (g)	Fiber (g)	NETT CHO (g)	CHO Count
Apple, big	64	1/2 Big	8	2	9	½
Apricot, dried	13	-	10		10	½
Avocado fruit	27	-		2	1	0
Banana, poovam	38	1/2 Medium	9	1	10	½
Banana, ripe, red	36	-	9	1	10	½
BlackBerry (Jamun)	74	12–15 no	8	3	10	½
Cherries, red	67	-	8	1	9	½

(Contd.)

FRUITS						
Fruits	Raw Weight (g) / 40 kcal	Portion Size	CHO (g)	Fiber (g)	NETT CHO (g)	CHO Count
Custard apple	40	1 Medium	8	2	9	½
Dates, processed	14	2 no	10	1	11	1
Fig	49	-	8	2	12	1
Gooseberry	170	-	7	13	14	1
Grapes, seeded, round, green	72	18-20 no	9	1	10	½
Grapes, seeded, round, black	66	-	9	1	10	½
Guava, pink flesh	86	-	8	6	11	1
Guava, white flesh	123	1 Medium	6	11	12	1
Jackfruit, ripe	55	3 no	8	2	9	½
Litchi	75	-	9	1	10	½
Mango, Ripe, Banganapalli	100	1 Medium	8	2	9	½
Muskmelon, orange flesh	173	4-5 Slices	7	3	9	½
Orange Pulp	107	1 Medium	8	1	9	½
Papaya, ripe	167	4 Thin long slices	8	5	11	1
Pear	106	1 Medium	9	5	12	1
Pineapple	93	1 Thick Slice	9	3	11	1
Plum	70	5 no	8	1	9	½
Sapota	54	1/2 Big	8	5	11	1
Strawberry	164	-	6	4	8	½
Lime Sweet, pulp	148	-	8	3	10	½
Tamarind, pulp	14	3tsp	9	1	10	½
Watermelon, dark green	195	1 Big slice	8	1	9	½

MILK AND MILK PRODUCTS

Milk and Milk Products	Raw Weight (g/ml)	Quantity	CHO (g)	Fiber (g)	NETT CHO (g)	CHO Count
Buttermilk (cow's milk)*	100 ml	1/2cup	2.5	0	2.5	0
Curd, cow's milk*	100 g	1/2cup	3	0	3	0
Milk, buffalo's	100 ml	1/2cup	8	0	8	½
Milk, cow's	100 ml	1/2cup	5	0	5	0
Paneer, cow's milk	100 g	-	12	0	12	1
Skimmed milk powder (cow's milk)*	100 g	-	51	0	51	3 ½
Skimmed milk, liquid*	100 ml	1/2cup	4	0	4	0

CONDIMENTS AND SPICES

Condiments And Spices	Raw Weight (g)	CHO (g)	Fiber (g)	NETT CHO (g)	CHO Count
Onion, big	100	10	2	11	1
Onion, small	100	10	1	11	1

NUTS

Nuts	Raw Weight (g) Per 85 kcal	Portion Size	CHO (g)	Fiber (g)	NETT CHO (g)	CHO Count
Almond	14	12 no		2	1	0
Cashew nut	14.5	6 no	4	1	5	0
Coconut, kernel, fresh	20	4tspn	1	2	2	0
Groundnut	16	20 no	3	2	4	0
Pistachio nut	15	23 no	2	2	3	0
Walnut	12	5 no	1	1	2	0

SUGARS						
Sugars	Raw Weight (g)	Cooked Portion	CHO (g)	Fiber (g)	NETT CHO (g)	CHO Count
Honey*	25	-	20	0	20	1
Jaggery(cane)	25	-	21	0	21	1½
Jaggery(date palm)*	25	-	22	0	22	1½
Refined sugar**	25	-	25	0	25	1½
Sago*	25	1 Cup	22	0	22	1½

Source: Carbohydrate counting calculations based on nutritional information from IFCT 2017

Note:

- Since the CHO content for marine foods, meat & poultry, and fats & oils are below detectable amounts, the CHO count for these exchanges considers zero.
- NETT CHO = (Carbohydrate per serving + Fibre per serving) – Fibre per serving ÷2
- Nutrient values have been rounded off to the nearest number
- * National Institute of Nutrition (NIN)
- ** Nutritive Value of Foods, U.S Department of Agriculture (USDA)
- Quantity as per food exchange list
- CHO – Carbohydrates
- g – grams
- ml – milli litre

References

1. Longvah, T., Ananthan, R., Bhaskarachary, K., &Venkaiah, K. (2017). *Indian Food Composition Tables,* India, Hyderabad: National Institute of Nutrition.
2. * Gopalan, C., Sastri, B .V.R..,&Balasubramanian, S. C. (1989). *Nutritive Value of Indian Foods (Rev.ed.).* India, Hyderabad: National Institute of Nutrition.
3. ** Susan, E., Gebhardt.,Robin, G., &Thomas. (2002). *Nutritive Value of Foods,* U.S Department of Agriculture.

Carbohydrate Counting (Continued…)

CARBOHYDRATE COUNTING OF SELECTED PACKAGED AND PROCESSED FOODS

MILK AND MILK PRODUCTS

Milk and Milk Products	Quantity (ml)	Serving Size (ml)	CHO (g) / 100 ml	FIBER (g) / 100 ml	NETT CHO (g) / 100 ml	CHO Count
Aavin milk 1.5 %	100	As desired	5	0	5	0
Aavin milk 3 %	100	As desired	5	0	5	0
Aavin milk 4 1/2 %	100	As desired	5	0	5	0
Aavin milk 6 %	100	As desired	5	0	5	0
Amul tazza (toned milk)	100	As desired	5	0	5	0
Arokya 4 1/2 %	100	As desired	5	0	5	0
Cavin stoned milk	100	As desired	4	0	4	0
Nestle a+ nourish	100	As desired	5	0	5	0
Nestle a+ slim	100	As desired	5	0	5	0
Niligiris 6 %	100	As desired	5	0	5	0
Niligiris toned milk 3 %	100	As desired	5	0	5	0
Tirumala 4 1/2 %	100	As desired	5	0	5	0
Milky mist unsweetened khoa	100	As desired	25	0	25	1½

Curd	Quantity	Serving Size	CHO (g) / 100 ml	FIBER (g) / 100 ml/g	NETT CHO (g) / 100 ml	CHO Count
Amul lassi	100 ml	As desired	13 ml	0	13	1
Amul spiced buttermilk	100 ml	As desired	2 ml	0	2	0
Cavin's curd	100 g	As desired	6 g	0	6	½
Epigamia greek yoghurt (natural)	100 g	90 g	6 g	0	6	0
Yakult yoghurt	100 g	65 g	18 g	0	18	1

Source: Nutritional Information from the Nutritional Label of the Packaged Food Products

Butter	Quantity (g)	Serving Size (g)	CHO (g) / 100 g	FIBER (g) / 100 g	NETT CHO (g)/ 100 g	CHO Count
Aavin cooking butter	100	As desired	0	0	0	0
Amul butter (salted)	100	As desired	0	0	0	0
Amul butter (unsalted)	100	As desired	0	0	0	0

Ghee	Quantity (g)	Serving Size (g)	CHO (g) / 100 g	FIBER (g) / 100 g	NETT CHO (g) / 100 g	CHO Count
Amul ghee	100	As desired	0	0	0	0
Milky mist ghee	100	As desired	0	0	0	0

Cheese	Quantity (g)	Serving Size (g)	CHO (g) / 100 g	FIBER (g) / 100 g	NETT CHO (g)/ 100 g	CHO Count
Amul cheese cubes	100	25	2	0	2	0
Amul cheese slice	100	20	1	0	1	0
Amul cheese spread	100	As desired	13	0	13	1
Britannia cheese	100	As desired	4	0	4	0

Paneer	Quantity (g)	Serving Size (g)	CHO (g) / 100 g	FIBER (g) / 100 g	NETT CHO (g) / 100 g	CHO Count
Milky mist paneer	100	As desired	5	0	5	0

Cream	Quantity (ml)	Serving Size (ml)	CHO (g) / 100 ml	FIBER (g) / 100 ml	NETT CHO (g)/ 100 ml	CHO Count
Amul fresh cream	100	As desired	3	0	3	0

Icecreams	Quantity (ml)	Serving Size (ml)	CHO (g) / 100 ml	FIBER (g) / 100 ml	NETT CHO (g) / 100 ml	CHO Count
Baskin Robins (vanilla)	100	As desired	21	0	21	1½
Feast (choco bar)	100	55	24	2	25	1½
Kwality walls Alphonso mango	100	48	23	1	24	1½
Kwality walls butterscotch	100	54	30	0	30	2
Kwality walls chocolate	100	53	26	1	27	2
Kwality walls cornetto (black forest)	100	75	37	5	40	2 ½
Kwality walls strawberry	100	53	23	2	24	1½
Kwality walls strawberry cheesecake	100	60	31	2	32	2
Kwality walls tutti fruit	100	51	23	3	25	1½
Kwality walls vanilla	100	53	23	2	24	1½
Magnum classic	100	70	29	1	30	2

Condensed Milk	Quantity (g)	Serving Size (g)	CHO (g) / 100 g	FIBER (g) / 100 g	NETT CHO (g) / 100 g	CHO Count
Nestle milkmaid	100	15	58	0	58	3 ½

Confectionery	Quantity (g)	Serving Size (g)	CHO (g) / 100 g	FIBER (g)/ 100 g	NETT CHO (g) / 100 g	CHO Count
Milky mist shrikhand	100	As desired	40	0	40	2½

Milkshakes	Quantity (ml)	SERVING SIZE (ml)	CHO (g) / 100 ml	FIBER (g) / 100 ml	NETT CHO (g) / 100 ml	CHO Count
Aavin badam milkshake	100	As desired	14	0	14	1
Aavin vanilla milkshake	100	As desired	13	0	13	1
Amul cool café	100	As desired	12	0	12	1
Cavin's chocolate milkshake	100	As desired	17	0	17	1
Nescafe chilled latte	100	As desired	11	0	11	1

Source: Nutritional Information from the Nutritional Label of the packaged Food Products

PROPRIETARY DRINKS

Proprietary Drinks	Quantity (g)	Serving Size (g)	CHO (g) / 100 g	FIBER (g) / 100 g	NETT CHO (g) / 100 g	CHO Count
Boost	100	20	82	3	84	5½
Bourn vita	100	20	85	4	87	5½
Complan	100	As desired	62	0	62	4½
Horlicks	100	27	79	0	79	5½
Horlicks lite	100	As desired	74	0	74	4½
Manna badam mix	100	As desired	87	0	87	5½
Manna Dates Rich (6months +)	100	As desired	74	0	74	4½
Manna health mix	100	As desired	75	6	78	5½
Manna ragi malt	100	As desired	87	0	87	5½
Manna rice rich (6 months +)	100	As desired	80	0	80	5½
Aavinbadam mix powder	100	As desired	85	0	85	5½

ENTERAL SUPPLEMENTS

Diabetic Supplements	Quantity (g)	Serving Size (g)	CHO (g) / 100 g	FIBER (g) / 100 g	NETT CHO (g) / 100 g	CHO Count
D- Protein	100	30	58	7	62	4 ½
Essential DM	100	50	61	3	63	4 ½
Fresubin DM	100	50	44	7	48	3 ½
Ensure Diabetes Care	100	52	60	5	63	4 ½ 9
Pentasure DLS	100	42	56	0	56	3 ½
Pentasure DM	100	20	62	6	65	4 ½
Prohance – D	100	50	46	8	50	3 ½
Resource diabetic	100	50	51	5	54	3 ½

Source: Nutritional Information from the Nutritional Label of the Packaged Food Products

Renal Supplements	Quantity (g)	Serving Size (g)	CHO (g) / 100 g	FIBER (g) / 100 g	NETT CHO (g) / 100 g	CHO Count
Essential Renal	100	25	66	0	66	4 ½
Fresubin HP	100	42	48	2	49	3 ½
Fresubin LP	100	21	60	3	62	4 ½
KabiPro	100	24	41	5	44	3
Nepro HP	100	89	44	3	46	3 ½
Nepro LP	100	87	52	3	54	3 ½
Pentasure Renal	100	21	67	0	67	4 ½
Resource Renal	100	50	60	4	62	4 ½
Resource Dialysis	100	50	48	4	50	3 ½

INSTANT CEREALS						
Instant Cereals	Quantity (g)	Serving Size (g)	CHO (g) / 100 g	FIBER (g) / 100 g	NETT CHO (g)/ 100 g	CHO Count
Horlicks oats	100	35	66	11	72	4½
Kellogg's chocos	100	30	84	5	87	5½
Kellogg's cornflakes	100	30	87	3	89	5½
Kellogg'smuseli	100	40	81	4	83	5½
Kellogg's special	100	30	85	0	85	5½
Modern bread atta shakti	100	As desired	52	5	55	3½
Modern enriched sweet bread	100	As desired	55	0	55	3½
Modern multigrain superseed	100	As desired	47	0	47	3½
Modern pav	100	As desired	51	0	51	3½
Modern sweet bun	100	As desired	56	0	56	3½
Modern whole wheat bread	100	As desired	47	6	50	3½
Quaker Oats	100	40	69	10	74	4½
Saffola masala oats	100	39	69	8	73	4½

Source: Nutritional Information from the Nutritional Label of the packaged Food Products

BAKERY PRODUCTS

BISCUITS						
Biscuits	Quantity (g)	Serving Size (g)	CHO (g) / 100 g	FIBER (g) / 100 g	NETT CHO (g)/ 100 g	CHO Count
50-50	100	As Desired	71	0	71	4½
Bourbon	100	As Desired	72	0	72	4½
Britannia rusk	100	As Desired	79	0	79	5½
Dark fantasy	100	As Desired	64	0	64	4½
Good day cashew	100	As Desired	63	0	63	4 ½
Good day chocolate	100	As Desired	71	0	71	4½
Good day pista	100	As Desired	65	0	65	4 ½
Hide N Seek	100	As Desired	73	0	73	4½
Jimjam	100	As Desired	73	0	73	4½
Little hearts	100	37	70	0	70	4½
Marie gold	100	As Desired	77	0	77	5½
Milk bikis	100	As Desired	75	0	75	5
Milk bikis milky sandwich	100	As Desired	68	0	68	4½
Nice time	100	As Desired	76	0	76	5½
Nutri choice digestive	100	As Desired	68	6	71	4½
Oreo	100	As Desired	71	0	71	4½
Parle G	100	As Desired	78	0	78	5½
Sunfeast marie light	100	As Desired	76	5	79	5 ½
Sunfeast marie light oats	100	As Desired	77	5	80	5 ½
Sunfeast marie light orange	100	As Desired	75	3	77	5 ½
Unibic	100	As Desired	68	0	68	4½
Waffy choco rolls	100	As Desired	76	0	76	5½
Waffy vanilla	100	As Desired	66	0	66	4 ½

Source: Nutritional Information from the Nutritional Label of the packaged Food Products

CAKES

Cakes	Quantity (g)	Serving Size (g)	CHO (g) / 100 g	FIBER (g) / 100 g	NETT CHO (g)/ 100 g	CHO Count
Britannia cake	100	60	55	0	55	3½
Britannia strawberry mufills	100	35	50	0	50	3½
Monginis swiss roll	100	40	58	0	58	3½
Lotte choco pie	100	28	57	0	57	3½

CHOCOLATES

Chocolates	Quantity (g or ml)	Serving Size (g or ml)	CHO (g) / 100 g	FIBER (g) / 100 g	NETT CHO (g) / 100 g	CHO Count
Bourneville rich cocoa	100	22	56	1	57	3½
Dairy milk chocolate	100	72	65	4	67	4½
Dairy milk crackle	100	11	54	2	55	3½
Dairy milk fruit and nut	100	34	61	2	62	4 ½
Dairy milk silk	100	37	58	0	58	3½
Dairy milk silk (caramello)	100	80	58	7	62	4½
Dairy milk silk (roasted almonds)	100	60	62	2	63	4½
Dairy milk silk oreo	100	60	63	1	64	4½
Ferro Rocher	100	As desired	60	2	61	4½
Gems	100	As desired	90	0	90	6
Kinder Joy	100	20	59	3	61	4½
Lickables	100	As desired	44	0	44	2½
Mentos	100	20	57	0	57	3½
Milky bar	100	As desired	70	0	70	4½
Nestle Kit Kat	100	18	61	1	62	4½
Nestle munch	100	As desired	65	1	66	4½
Nuttiest	100	60	48	3	50	3½

(Contd.)

CHOCOLATES

Chocolates	Quantity (g or ml)	Serving Size (g or ml)	CHO (g) / 100 g	FIBER (g) / 100 g	NETT CHO (g) / 100 g	CHO Count
Snickers	100	As desired	79	2	80	5 ½
Temptations rum raisins	100	As desired	74	0	74	4 ½
5 star	100	55	54	3	56	3 ½

BEVERAGES

Beverages	Quantity (ml)	Serving Size (ml)	CHO (g) / 100 ml	FIBER (g) / 100 ml	NETT CHO (g) / 100 ml	CHO Count
Appy	100	As desired	16	0	16	1
Bovonto	100	As desired	11	0	11	1
Coca-Cola	100	As desired	11	0	11	1
Fanta	100	As desired	13	0	13	1
Frooti	100	As desired	16	0	16	1
Gatorade	100	As desired	6	0	6	½
Glucovita(Lime)	100	As desired	92	0	92	6½
Limca	100	As desired	11	0	11	1
Maaza	100	As desired	14	0	14	1
Minute maid pulpy orange	100	As desired	13	0	13	1
Miranda	100	As desired	14	0	14	1
Mountain dew	100	As desired	12	0	12	1
Pink health cocoma	100	As desired	7	0	7	½
Real fruit juice mix	100	As desired	14	0	14	1
Red bull	100	As desired	11	0	11	1
Sprite	100	As desired	12	0	12	1
Thumbs up	100	As desired	10	0	10	½
Tropicana (Litchi)	100	As desired	14	0	14	1
Tropicana slice	100	As desired	17	0	17	1

Source: Nutritional Information from the Nutritional Label of the packaged Food Products

PROCESSED SNACKS

Processed Snacks	Quantity (g)	Serving Size (g)	CHO (g) / 100 g	FIBER (g) / 100 g	NETT CHO (g) / 100 g	CHO Count
Haldirams aloo bhuja	100	As desired	46	1	47	3 ½
Haldirams bhujia sev	100	As desired	37	1	38	2 ½
Haldirams moong dal	100	As desired	51	2	52	3 ½
Kurkure	100	As desired	54	0	54	3 ½
Corn puffs	100	As desired	73	1	74	4 ½
Lays	100	As desired	52	0	52	3 ½

SPREADS

Spreads	Quantity (g)	Serving Size (g)	CHO (g) / 100 g	FIBER (g) / 100 g	NETT CHO (g) / 100 g	CHO Count
Dr. Oetkar eggless sandwich spread	100	As desired	16	0	16	1
Fun foods peanut butter chocolate	100	As desired	28	0	28	2
Fun foods veg mayonnaise	100	As desired	9	0	9	½
Hersheys chocolate syrup	100	39	62	0	62	4 ½
Hershey's spread	100	As desired	64	0	64	4 ½
Kissanmixed fruit jam	100	20	71	0	71	4 ½
Kissan orange marmalade	100	20	71	0	71	4 ½
Lion dates jam	100	As desired	88	0	88	5 ½
Lion dates syrup	100	As desired	76	6	79	5 ½
Nutella spread	100	15	58	0	58	3 ½
Nutella hazelnut spread	100	As desired	23	0	23	1 ½

Source: Nutritional Information from the Nutritional Label of the packaged Food Products

READY TO MAKE FOODS

Ready To Make Foods	Quantity (g)	Serving Size (g)	CHO (g) / 100 g	FIBER (g) / 100 g	NETT CHO (g)/ 100 g	CHO Count
Aachi lemon rice paste	100	As desired	18	0	18	1
Aachi Tomato garlic rice paste	100	As desired	9	0	9	½
Act II popcorn classic salted	100	As desired	61	11	67	4 ½
Betty Crocker fan cake mix	100	22	70	2	71	4 ½
Fresher Idiyappam	100	As desired	33	0	33	2
ID Chapathi	100	39	55	0	55	3 ½
ID Idly batter	100	As desired	26	0	26	2
Knorr sweet corn mix	100	11	69	3	71	4 ½
Knorr tomato soup mix	100	13	69	4	71	4 ½
Maggi atta masala noodles	100	75	61	6	64	4 ½
Maggi masala cup noodles	100	70	59	3	61	4 ½
Maggi pasta (cheese macaroni)	100	70	68	4	70	4 ½
Maggi two minutes noodles	100	70	64	4	66	4 ½
Manna soya nuggets	100	As desired	32	0	32	2
McCain aloo tikki	100	As desired	25	0	25	1 ½
McCain burger patty	100	As desired	29	0	29	2
McCain chilly garlic potato	100	As desired	23	0	23	1 ½
McCain French fries	100	As desired	22	0	22	1 ½
McCain Mini samosa	100	As desired	33	0	33	2
McCain Potato cheese shots	100	As desired	24	0	24	1 ½
McCain Smileys	100	As desired	28	0	28	2
McCain Veg fingers	100	As desired	26	0	26	2
McCain veg nuggets	100	As desired	25	0	25	1 ½
McCain Wedges	100	As desired	19	0	19	1

READY TO MAKE FOODS

Ready To Make Foods	Quantity (g)	Serving Size (g)	CHO (g) / 100 g	FIBER (g) / 100 g	NETT CHO (g)/ 100 g	CHO Count
Modern Whole wheat parota	100	As desired	43	7	47	3 ½
Mother's Recipe ginger garlic paste	100	16	21	0	21	1 ½
MTR Bajji Bonda mix	100	25	59	1	60	4
MTR Dal Makani	100	150	12	0	12	1
MTR Gulab jamun	100	25	60	0	60	4
MTR Multigrain dosa	100	45	66	0	66	4 ½
MTR PalakPaneer	100	150	5	0	5	0
MTR Paneer butter masala	100	150	4	0	4	0
MTR Paneer makhani	100	150	9	0	9	½
MTR Pongal	100	150	10	0	10	½
MTR Ragi Dosa	100	45	65	0	65	4 ½
MTR Rava dosai	100	45	73	4	75	5
MTR Rava Idli	100	40	29	4	31	2
MTR Rice Idli	100	40	67	7	71	4 ½
MTR Sambar rice	100	150	12	0	12	1
MTR Tomato rice	100	125	14	0	14	1
MTR Upma	100	70	68	4	70	4 ½
MTR Vada	100	As desired	55	10	60	4
MTR Veg pulao	100	125	21	0	21	1 ½
MTR Vermicelli Kheer	100	As desired	86	0	86	5 ½
Pillsbury Eggless cooker cake	100	As desired	76	0	76	5 ½
Sunfeast Pasta treat (Tomato)	100	70	71	0	71	4 ½
Yipee Classic masala noodles	100	As desired	62	0	62	4 ½

Source: Nutritional Information from the Nutritional Label of the packaged Food Products

READY TO EAT FOODS

Ready To Eat Foods	Quantity (g)	Serving Size (g)	CHO (g) / 100 g	FIBER (g) / 100 g	NETT CHO (g) / 100 g	CHO Count
Haldiram's Gulab Jamun	100	26	68	0	68	4 ½
Haldiram's Rosogulla	100	26	58	0	58	3 ½
Haldiram's Son papdi	100	As desired	59	0	59	3 ½

READY TO MIX FOODS

Ready To Mix Foods	Quantity (g)	Serving Size (g)	CHO (g) / 100 g	FIBER (g) / 100 g	NETT CHO (g) / 100 g	CHO Count
Bambino Gulab jamun	100	As desired	63	0	63	4 ½
Cadbury Hot chocolate	100	20	86	10	91	6 ½
Hapima Fried rice mix	100	As desired	44	0	44	2 ½
Maggi Coconut powder	100	As desired	21	0	21	1 ½
Weikfield Caramel pudding	100	As desired	81	0	81	5 ½
Weikfield Custard powder	100	As desired	88	0	88	5 ½
Weikfield Falooda Mix	100	As desired	71	0	71	4 ½
Weikfield Jelly crystals	100	As desired	93	0	93	6 ½

Source: Nutritional Information from the Nutritional Label of the Packaged Food Products

MISCELLANEOUS FOODS

Miscellaneous	Quantity (g)	Serving Size (g)	CHO (g) / 100 g	FIBER (g) / 100 g	NETT CHO (g) / 100 g	CHO Count
Bindu Appalam	100	As desired	55	0	55	3 ½
Dabur Coconut Milk	100	As desired	4	0	4	0
Dabur honey	100	As desired	80	0	80	5 ½
DaburTomato Puree	100	As desired	7	0	7	½
Dr. Oetkar Chilli Sauce	100	As desired	36	0	36	2 ½
Dr. Oetkar Soya Sauce	100	As desired	21	0	21	1 ½
Kissan Ketchup	100	15	33	0	33	3
Kissan Mixed Fruit Squash	100	50	53	0	53	3 ½
Maggi Coconut Powder	100	As desired	21	0	21	1 ½
Mother's Recipe Punjabi Masala Pappad	100	As desired	43	0	43	2 ½
Ruchi Lime Pickle	100	As desired	9	0	9	½
Ruchi Mango Avvakai Pickle	100	As desired	10	0	10	½

CHO – Carbohydrates

g – Grams

ml – Milliliter

0 – Not Expressed

Source: Nutritional Information from the Nutritional Label of the Packaged Food Products

CARBOHYDRATE COUNTING – COOKED FOODS

Bajaj.M, Kothari.S, & Sherene.G

Tamil Nadu Government Multi Super Speciality Hospital, Chennai (2018)

Breads: 15 g Carb (1 carb)	Starchy Vegetables: 15 g carb
1 Slice bread, white, wheat or whole grain	1/3 C plantain green
1 Small pau/dinner roll	½ C potato sabji*
½ Roti (bajra, makai, jowar)	1 Small potato, boiled or baked
1 Chapati, 6" diameter	½ Potatoes, mashed
¾ Paratha or thepla, 6"*	½ C sweet potatoes
½ Paneer paratha	½ C peas
¾ Potato paratha, 6"*	½ C corn
1/4th of 8"X 2" Naan	½ C yam
2 Puris 5"	French fries*
1 Dosaapproximately 10" diameter	1c Mixed veg (corn, peas)
1 Small idli	
2 Mini ravaidlis	
25g/3tbsp Atta(Whole Wheat)	
25 G/ 3tbsp Maida (All-Purpose flour)	

Cereals/grains: 15 g Carb (1 carb)	Pulses/dals/beans: 15 g Carb
½ C Poha (aval uppuma)	½ C Lentils, cooked
½ C Dalia (cooked)	½ C Toor dal, cooked
½ C Upma (cooked)	½ C Mung dal, cooked
½ C Pasta (cooked)	1C Thin mixed dal, cooked
½ C Cooked hot cereal	½ C Kidney beans, cooked
1/3 C White rice cooked	½ C Chickpeas, cooked
1/3 C Brown rice cooked	½ C Lobia(black-eyed peas) cooked
1/3 C Tamarind rice	1/3 C Besan
1/3 C BisibhelaBhath	1 C Rasam
½ C Biryani/pulao*meat	½ C Sambar
½ C Khichadi/khichri, cooked	½ C Vegetable korma
1 Square dhokla	1 C Aloogobhi
½ C Aviyal	1 C Sprouted moong salad
1/3 C Uppuma	1 ¼ C Chicken curry
½ Uttapam vegetable(small) or	1 ¼ C Chicken Chettinad curry
1 mini Uttapam, 4"	

Sweets: 15 g Carb (limit to 10% of diet)	Milk/yogurt: 15 g Carb
2 Nankhatai, small*	0.1% Skim milk -220ml
1 Small Gulab Jamoon*	6.5%, Whole milk*-300ml
1/3 C Carrot halwa*	4% Milk-340ml
¼ C Soojihalwa*	
½ C kulfi*	
½ Small laddoo	
1 Medium rosogullah	
1 Small ras malai	
¼ C Shrikand	
½ C Ice cream*	
1 Small cupcake unfrosted*	
2 Small cookies, plain	
1 tbsp honey	
1 tbsp sugar	

Snack foods: 15 g Carb (1 Carb Choice)	Combination foods/Misc: 30 g Carbs (2CHO Servings)
1oz. Bhelpuri	1 C Meat & potato salan/curry*
1oz Chivda	1 C Haleem (made with wheat, lentils, meat)*
6 Panipuri	1 C Dal gosht*
2 Papad	1 C Kadhi* made with besan
¾ Veg samosa (1samosa=21g CHO)*	12 Chicken nuggets*
1 Medium vegetable cutlet*	1 C Macaroni & cheese*
3 pcs Pakoda spinach*	1(3"x4") piece of lasagna*
1 kachori(veg)*	¼ of 10-inch pizza*
1 kachori(mung dal*)	
2 pcs Cauliflower bhajia	Foods like sugar-free sodas and beverages,
2 pcs Dahivada*	artificial sweeteners, few spices, and seasonings
1oz. Banana chips	fall into this category.
3 C Popcorn	
2 Rice cakes 4"	
1 ½ C Mumbra(puffed rice)	
10 French fries*	

Vegetables: 5 g Carb (Count if serving size more than 15 g)	Fruits/Juices: 15g Carbs
½ C Cooked vegetables (asparagus, green	1 Small Apple
beans, bean sprouts, beets, broccoli, cabbage,	4 Whole apricots (fresh)
carrots, cauliflower, eggplant, okra, onions,	1 Small banana (4oz) or ½ medium
spinach, tomato, turnips, and zucchini etc.)	1 Medium Chiku(sapota)
1 C Raw vegetable	12 Sweet cherries
½ C Tomato or vegetable juice	3 Dates
¼ C Tomato puree	2 Medium figs fresh
½ C Tomato sauce	1 ½ Dried Figs
½ C Pasta	½ C Fruit cocktail
	½ Grapefruit
	17 Grapes
	6 Jambu
	1 Kiwi
	¾ C Mandarin oranges
	½ Small mango(½ C)
	½ C Canned peaches/pears
	1 Small orange
	1 C Papaya cubes
	½ Large pear or 1 small
	1 Medium peach
	¾ C Fresh pineapple
	2 Small plums
	3 Dried plums (prunes)
	3 tbsp raisins
	1 C Raspberries
	1 ¼ C Strawberries
	1 Medium seetaphal
	1 ¼ C Watermelon cubes
	½ C Apple juice

References

1. ADA complete guide to carbohydrate counting. (n.d). Retrieved from http://www. diabetes.org/food-and-fitness/food/what-can-ieat/understanding-carbohydrates/ carbohydrate-counting.html

2. Carbohydrate Counting for Traditional South Asian Foods. (n.d). Retrieved from http://www.sjsu.edu/people/ashwini.wagle/Southasians/Carbohydrate%20 Counting%20Tool%20for%20South%20Asians%204th%20Version.pdf

3. Gopalan, C., Sastri, B .V.R., & Balasubramanian, S. C. (1989). Nutritive Value of Indian Foods (Rev.ed.). India, Hyderabad: National Institute of Nutrition.

4. Holzmeister, L.A. (2010). The diabetes carbohydrate and fat gram guide. Academy of Nutrition and Dietetics (AND).

FAT PROTEIN UNIT

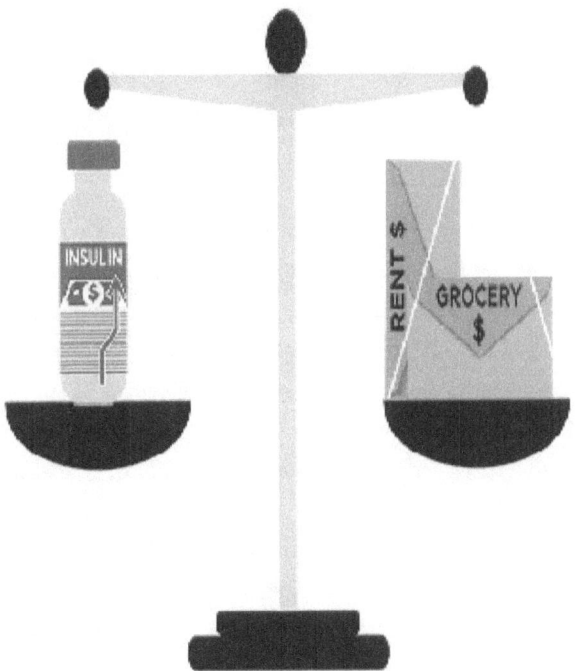

FAT PROTEIN UNIT (FPU)

Managing diabetes is not a science but an art which involves food and medicine. It is more important to understand the imbalance in our body's basic systems and restore balances, in addition to naming the disease and matching the pill to the ill. Carbohydrates, the predominant macronutrient affect the postprandial glycemic control and are the primary determinants for calculating mealtime insulin doses in type 1 diabetics.

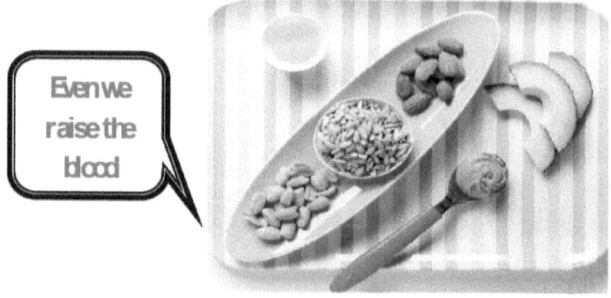

Emerging evidence from recent research and the use of continuous glucose monitoring have shown that other nutritional properties of food, including fat, protein, and glycemic index (GI), can significantly affect postprandial glucose excursions. Fat causes delayed hyperglycemia by 3–5 hours after eating and protein have an effect in 1.5 hours. Delayed postprandial glycemic response requires management in order to reduce the progression of already existing complications of diabetes. It mainly helps to prevent the micro and macrovascular complications of the disease. These findings highlight the need for alternative mealtime insulin dosing algorithm. (Bell, Toschi, Steil& Wolpert, 2016).

The new algorithm developed to handle the glycemic response due to fat protein in the meal consumed is

- The Warsaw Pump Therapy School (WPTS) or 'Warsaw' formula.

The Warsaw formula uses the usual Insulin to carbohydrate ratio to calculate the insulin dose for carbohydrate which is given as a normal dose before the meal. Additional insulin is calculated using a fat/protein unit

(FPU) where 1 unit of insulin is given for every 100kcal in the meal from fat and protein.

The additional insulin is given as an extended bolus over 3–6 hours, depending on the number of FPUs, using CSII.

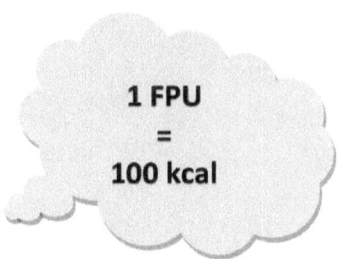

1 FPU
=
100 kcal

THE WARSAW FORMULA

SAMPLE CALCULATIONS	
Insulin: Carbohydrate ratio (ICR)	1:10 g
Meal carbohydrate	77g
Insulin = 77/ ICR= 77/10	7.7 units
Calories from fat and protein (672 minus 288 kcal)	384 kcal
1 fat/protein unit (FPU)	100 kcal
Total FPU	4
Additional units of insulin	4 units
Additional units are given as an extended bolus over 3–6 hours	

Hibbert-Jones (2016)

Note:

- For example a small size pizza provides 672 kcal
- Abbreviations: ICR – Insulin: Carbohydrate Ratio, CSII – Continuous Subcutaneous Insulin Infusion

References

- Bell, J.K., Toschi, E., Steil, G.M., & Wolpert, A.H. (2016).Optimized Mealtime Insulin Dosing for Fat and Protein in Type 1 Diabetes: Application of a Model-Based Approach to Derive Insulin Doses for Open-Loop Diabetes Management. *Diabetes Care, 39*,1631-1634.
- Hibbert-Jones, E.(2016).Fat and protein counting in type 1 diabetes, *Diabetes Care*, 33(7).

FAT PROTEIN UNIT (FPU)

Bajaj, M., Sherene, G., & Kothari, S.

Tamil Nadu Government Multi Super Speciality Hospital, Chennai (2018)

CEREALS

Cereals	Quantity (g)	Serving Size (g)	Protein (g) / 100 g	FAT (g) / 100 g	Fat Protein Calories (Kcal)	Fat Protein Unit
Barley	100	25	10.94	1.30	55	1
Chapathi, whole wheat flour(dry)	100	25	10.57	1.53	56	1
Dosa flour (dry)	100	25	12.00	0.00	48	0
Idly flour (dry)	100	25	12.00	0.00	48	0
Quinoa	100	25	13.11	5.50	102	1
Rice, raw milled	100	25	7.94	0.52	36	0
Rice flakes (dry)	100	25	7.44	1.14	40	0
Rice, parboiled milled	100	25	7.81	0.55	36	0
Wheat vermicelli roasted	100	25	10.37	0.49	46	0
Wheat, vermicelli (dry)	100	25	9.70	0.45	43	0
Wheat flour, refined (dry)	100	25	10.36	0.76	48	0
Wheat, semolina (dry)	100	25	11.38	0.74	52	1

MILLETS

Millets	Quantity (g)	Serving Size (g)	Protein (g) / 100 g	Fat (g) / 100 g	Fat Protein Calories (Kcal)	Fat Protein Unit
Bajra	100	25	10.96	5.43	93	1
Jowar	100	25	9.97	1.73	55	1
Ragi	100	25	7.16	1.92	46	0
Samai	100	25	10.13	3.89	76	1
Varagu	100	25	8.92	2.55	59	1

Source: FPU values are based on nutritional information from IFCT 2017.

PULSES

Pulses	Quantity (g)	Serving Size (g)	Protein (g) / 100 g	Fat (g) / 100 g	Fat Protein Calories (kcal)	Fat Protein Unit
Bengal gram, dhal	100	25	21.55	5.31	134	1
Bengal gram, whole	100	25	18.77	5.11	121	1
Black gram, dhal	100	25	23.06	1.69	107	1
Black gram, whole	100	25	21.97	1.58	102	1
Cowpea, white	100	25	21.25	1.14	95	1
Green gram, dhal	100	25	23.88	1.35	108	1
Green gram, whole	100	25	22.53	1.14	100	1
Horse gram, whole	100	25	21.73	0.62	93	1
Peas dry	100	25	20.43	1.89	99	1
Rajma, red	100	25	19.91	1.77	96	1
Red gram, dhal	100	25	21.70	1.56	101	1
Soyabean, white	100	22.5	37.80	19.42	326	3

VEGETABLES – GREEN LEAFY VEGETABLES

Group A (Green Leafy Vegetables)	Quantity (g)	Serving Size (g)	Protein (g) / 100 g	Fat (g) / 100 g	Fat Protein Calories (kcal)	Fat Protein Unit
Agathi leaves	100	100	8.01	1.35	44	0
Amaranth leaves, green	100	100	3.29	0.65	19	0
Cabbage, green	100	50	1.36	0.12	7	0
Cauliflower leaves	100	200	3.90	0.42	19	0
Drumstick leaves	100	50	6.41	1.64	40	0
Fenugreek leaves	100	100	3.68	0.83	22	0
Lettuce	100	100	1.54	0.27	9	0
Mustard leaves	100	100	3.52	0.50	19	0
Ponnanganni	100	100	5.29	0.71	28	0
Radish leaves	100	150	2.22	0.51	13	0
Spinach	100	150	2.14	0.64	14	0

VEGETABLES – ROOTS AND TUBERS

Group B (Roots and Tubers)	Quantity (g)	Serving Size (g)	Protein (g) / 100 g	Fat (g) / 100 g	Fat Protein Calories (kcal)	Fat Protein Unit
Beetroot	100	140	1.95	0.14	9	0
Carrot, orange	100	150	0.95	0.47	8	0
Colocasia	100	60	3.31	0.17	15	0
Potato, brown skin big	100	70	1.54	0.23	8	0
Sweet potato, Pink skin	100	55	1.27	0.33	8	0
Tapioca	100	60	1.03	0.20	6	0
Yam, elephant	100	60	2.56	0.14	12	0

VEGETABLES – OTHER VEGETABLES

Group C (Other Vegetables)	Quantity (g)	Serving Size (g)	Protein (g) / 100 g	Fat (g) / 100 g	Fat Protein Calories (kcal)	Fat Protein Unit
Ash gourd	100	170	0.79	0.14	4	0
Beans scarlet, tender	100	70	2.86	0.99	20	0
Bitter gourd, jagged, teeth ridges, elongate	100	145	1.44	0.24	8	0
Bottle gourd, elongate, pale green	100	270	0.53	0.13	3	0
Brinjal all varieties	100	110	1.48	0.32	9	0
Cauliflower	100	130	2.15	0.44	13	0
Cucumber, green, elongate	100	150	0.71	0.16	4	0
Ladies finger	100	110	2.08	0.22	10	0
Plantain flower	100	140	1.47	0.63	12	0
Ridge gourd	100	230	0.91	0.14	5	0
Snake gourd, long, pale green	100	240	0.98	0.25	6	0
Tomato red ripe, local	100	150	0.90	0.47	8	0
Tomato, green	100	150	1.12	0.27	7	0
Zucchini, green	100	150	1.10	0.51	9	0

Source: FPU values are based on nutritional information from IFCT 2017.

FRUITS

Fruits	Quantity (g)	Serving Size (g)	Protein (g) / 100 g	Fat (g) / 100 g	Fat Protein Calories (kcal)	Fat Protein Unit
Apple, big	100	65	0.29	0.64	7	0
Banana, poovam	100	40	1.49	0.35	9	0
Custard apple	100	40	1.62	0.67	13	0
Dates, processed	100	14	1.18	0.41	8	0
Gooseberry	100	16	0.34	0.16	3	0
Grapes, green round seeded	100	70	0.77	0.29	6	0
Guava, white flesh	100	120	1.44	0.32	9	0
Jackfruit, ripe	100	55	2.74	0.15	12	0
Jambu fruit, ripe	100	70	0.82	0.17	5	0
Mango, ripe, banganapalli	100	100	0.54	0.55	7	0
Muskmelon, orange flesh	100	175	0.42	0.35	5	0
Orange Pulp	100	107	0.70	0.13	4	0
Papaya, ripe	100	167	0.42	0.16	3	0
Pear	100	106	0.36	0.27	4	0
Pineapple	100	100	0.52	0.16	4	0
Plum	100	60	0.64	0.40	6	0
Sapota	100	50	0.92	1.26	15	0
Strawberry	100	160	0.97	0.56	9	0
Sweet lime, pulp	100	100	0.76	0.20	5	0
Tamarind, pulp	100	20	2.92	0.15	13	0
Watermelon, dark green	100	200	0.60	0.16	4	0

Source: FPU values are based on nutritional information from IFCT 2017.

MILK AND MILK PRODUCTS

Milk Products	Quantity (g)	Serving Size (g)	Protein (g) / 100 g	Fat (g) / ml 100 g	Fat Protein Calories (kcal)	Fat Protein Unit
Buttermilk (Cow's Milk)*	100 ml	400 ml	0.80 ml	1.10 ml	13	0
Milk, whole, Buffalo	100 ml	100 ml	3.68 ml	6.58 ml	74	1
Milk, whole, Cow	100 ml	150 ml	3.26 ml	4.48 ml	53	1
Skimmed milk*	100 ml	225 ml	2.50 ml	0.10 ml	11	0
Curd*	100 g	125 g	3.10 g	4.00 g	48	0
Panner	100 g	40 g	18.86 g	14.78 g	208	2
Skimmed milk Powder*	100 g	18 g	38.00 g	0.10 g	153	2

MEAT AND POULTRY

Meat and Poultry	Quantity (g)	Serving Size (g)	Protein (g) / 100 g	Fat (g) / 100 g	Fat Protein Calories (kcal)	Fat Protein Unit
Beef, chops	100	60	19.82	6.71	140	1
Chicken, poultry breast, skinless	100	50	21.81	9.00	168	2
Egg poultry, whole raw	100	50	13.28	9.15	135	1
Goat, chops	100	65	20.39	5.98	135	1

MARINE FOODS

Marine Products	Quantity (g)	Serving Size (g)	Protein (g) / 100 g	Fat (g) / 100 g	Fat Protein Calories (kcal)	Fat Protein Unit
Anchovy (Nethili)	100	50	19.88	0.78	87	1
Paarai (Jackfish)	100	50	21.58	1.84	103	1
Pomfret, black	100	50	18.91	4.83	119	1
Prawns, big	100	90	19.24	0.52	82	1
Salmon fish	100	50	20.97	9.86	173	2
Vanjaram (Seer fish)	100	50	22.28	5.18	136	1

Source: FPU values are based on nutritional information from IFCT 2017.

FATS

Fats	Quantity (g)	Serving Size (g)	Protein (g) / 100 g	Fat (g) / 100 g	Fat Protein Calories (kcal)	Fat Protein Unit
Butter *	100 g	10 g	0.00 g	81.00 g	729	7
Ghee, Cow *	100 g	10 g	0.00 g	100.00 g	900	9
Oil *	100 ml	10 ml	0.00 ml	100.00 ml	900	9

NUTS AND OILSEEDS

Nuts and Oilseeds	Quantity (g)	Serving Size (g)	Protein (g) / 100 g	Fat (g) / 100 g	Fat Protein Calories (kcal)	Fat Protein Unit
Almond	100	14	18.41	58.49	600	6
Cashew nut	100	15	18.78	45.20	482	5
Coconut, Kernel, Fresh	100	21	3.84	41.38	388	4
Groundnut	100	16	23.65	39.63	451	5
Mustard seed	100	3	19.51	40.19	440	4
Pistachio nut	100	15	23.35	42.49	476	5
Walnut	100	13	14.92	64.27	638	6

Source: FPU values are based on nutritional information from IFCT 2017.

Note:

- Nutrient values have been rounded off to the nearest number
- FPU #(AS PER FOOD EXCHANGE LIST)
- Abbreviations: G - Gram

References

1. Longvah, T., Ananthan, R., Bhaskarachary, K., &Venkaiah, K. (2017). Indian Food Composition Tables, National Institute of Nutrition.
2. * Gopalan, C., Sastri, B .V. R, &Balasubramanian, S. C. (2012). Nutritive Value of Indian Foods, National Institute of Nutrition.
3. ** Susan, E., Gebhardt., Robin, G., & Thomas. (2002). Nutritive Value of Foods, U.S Department of Agriculture.

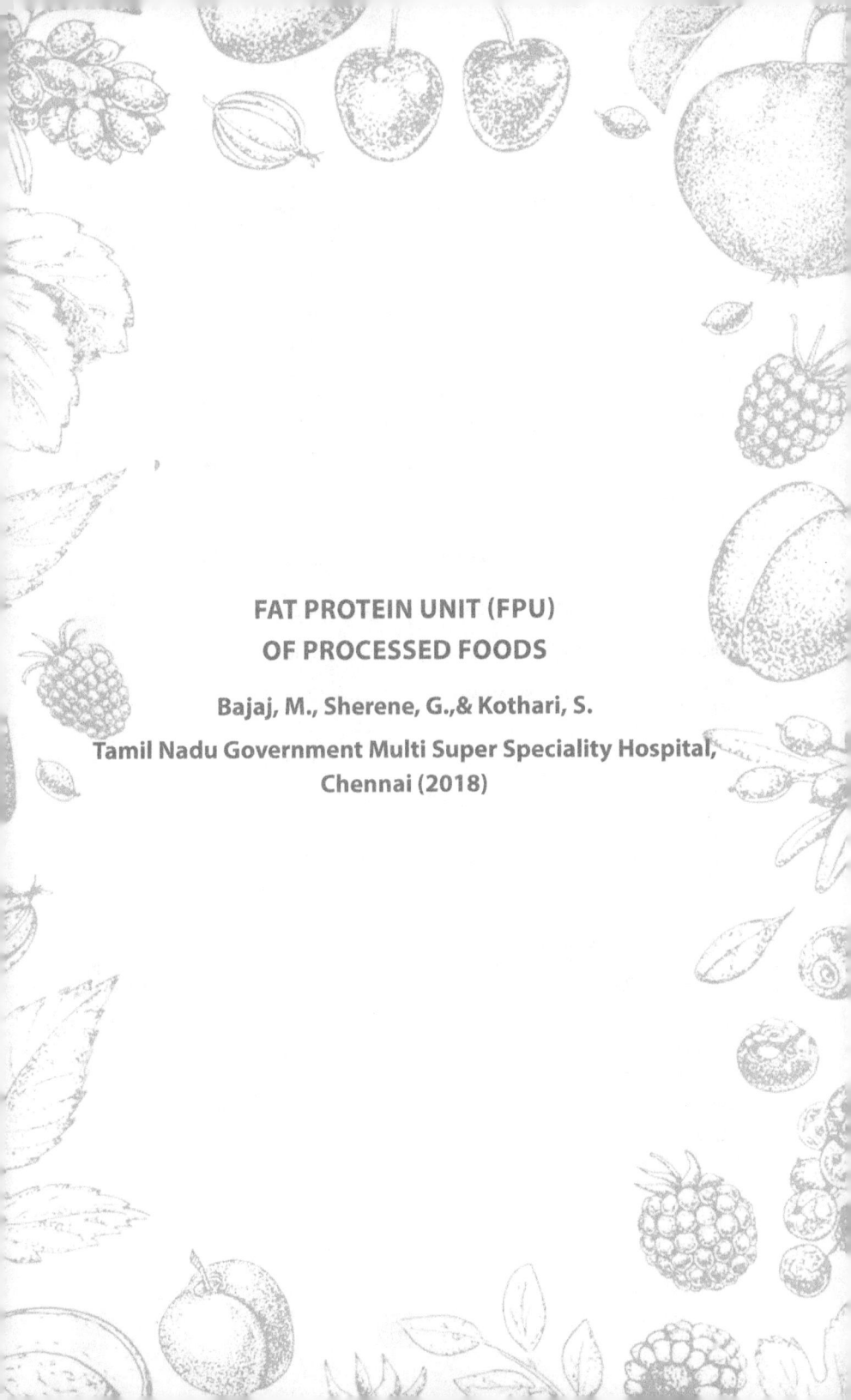

FAT PROTEIN UNIT (FPU)
OF PROCESSED FOODS

Bajaj, M., Sherene, G.,& Kothari, S.

Tamil Nadu Government Multi Super Speciality Hospital,
Chennai (2018)

¹ 1 Fat Protein Unit (FPU) = 100 Kcal

MILK AND MILK PRODUCTS

Milk and Milk Products	Quantity (g)	Serving Size (g)	Protein (g) / 100 ml	FAT (g) / 100 ml	Fat Protein Calories (Kcal)	Fat protein unit (FPU)
Aavin 1.5%	100	As Desired	3.40	1.50	27	0
Aavin 3%	100	As Desired	3.20	3.00	40	0
Aavin 4.5%	100	As Desired	3.20	4.50	53	1
Aavin 6%	100	As Desired	3.40	6.00	68	1
Amul tazza (Toned Milk)	100	As Desired	3.00	3.00	39	0
Arokya 4.5%	100	As Desired	3.00	4.50	53	1
Cavins Toned Milk	100	As Desired	3.24	1.60	27	0
Nestle A+ Nourish	100	As Desired	3.00	3.00	39	0
Nestle A+ Slim	100	As Desired	3.00	0.20	14	0
Nilgiris 6%	100	As Desired	3.40	6.00	68	1
Nilgris Toned Milk 3%	100	As Desired	3.20	3.00	40	0
Sofit Soya Milk	100	As Desired	3.20	2.00	31	0
Tirumala 4.5%	100	As Desired	3.25	4.50	54	1
Milky Mist Unsweetened Khoa	100	As Desired	16.30	22.00	263	3

Curd	Quantity (g)	Serving Size (g)	Protein (g) / 100 ml	Fat (g) / 100 ml	Fat Protein Calories (Kcal)	Fat Protein Unit (FPU)
Amul lassi	100 ml	As Desired	2.30	2.00	27	0
Amul spiced buttermilk	100 ml	As Desired	1.70	2.00	25	0
Cavin's Curd	100 g	As Desired	3.70	3.00	42	0
Epigamia Greek Yoghurt (Natural)	100 g	90	8.21	2.56	56	1
Yakult Yoghurt	100 g	65	1.23	0.00	5	0

Source: Nutritional Information from the Nutritional Label of the Packaged Food Product

Butter	Quantity (g)	Serving Size (g)	Protein (g) / 100 g	Fat (g) / 100 g	Fat Protein Calories (Kcal)	Fat Protein Unit (FPU)
Aavin Cooking Butter	100	As Desired	1.00	82.00	742	7
Amul Butter (Salted)	100	As Desired	0.50	80.00	722	7
Amul Butter (Unsalted)	100	100	0.60	82.00	740	7

Ghee	Quantity (g)	Serving Size (g)	Protein (g) / 100 g	Fat (g) / 100 g	Fat Protein Calories (Kcal)	Fat Protein Unit (FPU)
Amul Ghee	100	As Desired	0.00	90.50	815	8
Milky Mist Ghee	100	As Desired	0.00	99.70	897	9
Amul Butter (Unsalted)	100	100	0.60	82.00	740	7

Cheese	Quantity (g)	Serving Size (g)	Protein (g) / 100 g	Fat (g) / 100 g	Fat Protein Calories (Kcal)	Fat Protein Unit (FPU)
Amul Cheese Cubes	100	25	20.00	26.00	314	3
Amul Cheese Slice	100	20	20.00	25.00	305	3
Amul Cheese Spread	100	As Desired	11.20	20.00	225	2
Britannia Cheese	100	As Desired	17.00	25.00	293	3

Paneer	Quantity (g)	Serving Size (g)	Protein (g) / 100 g	Fat (g) / 100 g	Fat Protein Calories (Kcal)	Fat Protein Unit (FPU)
Milky Mist Paneer	100	As Desired	16.10	22.00	262	3

Cream	Quantity (ml)	Serving Size (ml)	Protein (g) / 100 ml	Fat (g) / 100 ml	Fat Protein Calories (Kcal)	Fat Protein Unit (FPU)
Amul Fresh Cream	100	As Desired	2.00	25.00	233	2

Source: Nutritional Information from the Nutritional Label of the Packaged Food Product

Icecream	Quantity (ml)	Serving Size (ml)	Protein (g) / 100 ml	Fat (g) / 100 ml	Fat Protein Calories (Kcal)	Fat Protein Unit (FPU)
Baskin Robins (Vanilla)	100	As Desired	4.07	12.00	124	1
Feast (Chocobar)	100	55	3.09	19.00	183	2
Kwality Walls Alphonsa Mango	100	48	3.54	9.00	95	1
Kwality Walls Butterscotch	100	54	3.51	11.00	113	1
Kwality Walls Chocolate	100	53	3.58	10.75	111	1
Kwality Walls Cornetto (Black Forest)	100	75	4.40	17.00	171	2
Kwality Walls Strawberry	100	53	3.96	11.00	115	1
Kwality Walls Strawberry Cheesecake	100	60	3.33	7.00	76	1
Kwality Walls Tutti fruti	100	51	3.92	8.00	88	1
Kwality Walls Vanilla	100	53	4.00	11.29	118	1
Magnum Classic	100	70	4.14	20.00	197	2

Condensed Milk	Quantity (g)	Serving Size (g)	Protein (g) / 100 g	Fat (g) / 100 g	Fat Protein Calories (Kcal)	Fat Protein Unit (FPU)
Nestle Milkmaid	100	15	8.50	4.00	70	1

Confectionery	Quantity (g)	Serving Size (g)	Protein (g) / 100 g	Fat (g) / 100 g	Fat Protein Calories (Kcal)	Fat Protein Unit (FPU)
Milky Mist Shrikhand	100	As Desired	8.00	7.00	95	1

Source: Nutritional Information from the Nutritional Label of the Packaged Food Product

Milkshakes	Quantity (ml)	Serving Size (ml)	Protein (g) / 100 ml	Fat (g) / 100 ml	Fat Protein Calories (Kcal)	Fat Protein Unit (FPU)
Aavin Badam Milkshake	100	As Desired	2.90	3.00	39	0
Aavin Vanilla Milkshake	100	As Desired	3.00	3.00	39	0
Amul Cool Cafe	100	As Desired	3.50	5.00	59	1
Cavin's Chocolate Milk Shake	100	As Desired	3.40	3.00	41	0
Nescafe Chilled Latte	100	As Desired	2.90	3.00	39	0

PROPRIETARY DRINKS

Health Drinks	Quantity (g)	Serving Size (g)	Protein (g) / 100 g	Fat (g) / 100 g	Fat Protein Calories (Kcal)	Fat Protein Unit (FPU)
Aavin Badam Mix Powder	100	As Desired	5.00	4.00	56	1
Boost	100	20	7.50	2.50	53	1
Bourn Vita	100	20	7.00	2.00	46	0
Complan	100	As Desired	18.00	11.00	171	2
Horlicks	100	27	11.00	2.00	62	1
Horlicks Lite	100	As Desired	13.00	2.00	70	1
Manna Badam Mix	100	As Desired	8.91	0.89	44	0
Manna Dates Rich (6 Months +)	100	As Desired	15.32	1.21	72	1
Manna Health Mix	100	As Desired	11.00	1.00	53	1
Manna Ragi Malt	100	As Desired	8.60	0.92	43	0
Manna Rice Rich (6 Months +)	100	As Desired	15.66	1.05	72	1

Source: Nutritional Information from the Nutritional Label of the Packaged Food Product

ENTERAL SUPPLEMENTS

Diabetic	Quantity (g)	Serving Size (g)	Protein (g) / 100 g	Fat (g) / 100 g	Fat Protein Calories (Kcal)	Fat Protein Unit (FPU)
D- Protein	100	33	78.70	1.51	328	3
Essential DM	100	50	20.00	14.00	206	2
Fresubin DM	100	50	20.20	20.00	261	3
Ensure Diabetes Care	100	52	20.10	14.61	212	2
Pentasure DM	100	50	22.00	11.54	192	2
Pentasure DM	100	20	22.00	11.54	192	2
Prohance – D	100	50	20.20	19.20	254	3
Resource diabetic	100g	50	22	19	259	3

Renal	Quantity (g)	Serving Size (g)	Protein (g) / 100 g	Fat (g) / 100 g	Fat Protein Calories (Kcal)	Fat Protein Unit (FPU)
Essential renal	100	25	9.00	20.00	216	2
Fresubin HP	100	42	21.50	25.00	311	3
Fresubin LP	100	21	9.00	22.00	234	2
KabiPro	100	24	42.00	3.00	195	2
Nepro HP	100	89	21.61	25.60	317	3
Nepro LP	100	87	12.19	26.12	284	3
Pentasure DLS	100	42	18.00	24.70	294	3
Pentasure renal	100	21	9.00	17.30	192	2
Resource renal	100	50	12.00	20.00	228	2
Resource Dialysis	100	50	24.00	20.00	276	3

Source: Nutritional Information from the Nutritional Label of the Packaged Food Product

INSTANT CEREALS

Instant Cereals	Quantity (g)	Serving Size (g)	Protein (g) / 100 g	Fat (g) / 100 g	Fat Protein Calories (Kcal)	Fat Protein Unit (FPU)
Horlicks Oats	100	35	13.00	10.00	142	1
Kellogg's Chocos	100	30	9.00	1.00	45	0
Kellogg's Cornflakes	100	30	6.66	1.00	36	0
Kellogg's muesli	100	40	7.50	5.00	75	1
Kellogg's Special	100	30	8.33	1.00	42	0
Modern Bread Atta Shakthi	100	As Desired	9.80	2.50	62	1
Modern Enriched Sweet Bread	100	As Desired	7.20	2.71	53	1
Modern Pav	100	As Desired	8.00	2.30	53	1
Modern Sweet Bun	100	As Desired	8.60	1.14	45	0
Modern Whole Wheat Bread	100	As Desired	9.60	2.39	60	1
Quaker Oats	100	40	12.00	10.00	138	1
Saffola Masala Oats	100	39	11.50	7.00	109	1

Source: Nutritional Information from the Nutritional Label of the Packaged Food Product

BAKERY PRODUCTS

BISCUITS						
Biscuits	Quantity (g)	Serving Size (g)	Protein (g) / 100 g	Fat (g) / 100 g	Fat Protein Calories (Kcal)	Fat Protein Unit (FPU)
50-50	100	As Desired	7.00	20.00	208	2
Bourbon	100	As Desired	5.00	20.00	200	2
Britannia Rusk	100	As Desired	8.00	11.00	131	1
Dark Fantasy	100	As Desired	5.70	25.00	248	2
Good Day Cashew	100	As Desired	7.00	24.00	244	2
Good Day Chocolate	100	As Desired	5.00	21.00	209	2
Good Day Pista	100	As Desired	7.00	24.00	244	2
Hide N Seek	100	As Desired	5.90	18.00	186	2
Jim Jam	100	As Desired	5.00	19.00	191	2
Little Hearts	100	37	7.00	20.00	208	2
Marie Gold	100	As Desired	8.00	12.00	140	1
Milk Bikis	100	As Desired	7.00	14.00	154	2
Milk Bikis Milky Sandwich	100	As Desired	7.00	22.00	226	2
Nice Time	100	As Desired	6.00	15.00	159	2
Nutri Choice Digestive	100	As Desired	8.00	21.00	221	2
Oreo	100	As Desired	5.30	20.00	201	2
Parle G	100	As Desired	6.90	13.00	145	1
Sunfeast Marie Light	100	As Desired	8.30	13.10	151	2
Sunfeast Marie Light Oats	100	As Desired	8.90	11.00	135	1
Sunfeast Marie Light Orange	100	As Desired	9.40	13.60	160	2
Unibic	100	As Desired	5.50	21.00	211	2
Waffy Vanilla	100	As Desired	2.60	28.00	262	3

Source: Nutritional Information from the Nutritional Label of the Packaged Food Product

CAKES

Biscuits	Quantity (g)	Serving Size (g)	Protein (g) / 100 g	Fat (g) / 100 g	Fat Protein Calories (Kcal)	Fat Protein Unit (FPU)
Britannia Cake	100	60	6.00	20.00	204	2
Britannia Strawberry Mufills	100	35	4.00	18.00	178	2
Lotte Choco Pie	100	28	4.80	17.00	172	2
Monginis Swiss Roll	100	40	8.35	20.00	213	2
Waffy Choco Rolls	100	As desired	4.20	15.00	152	2

CHOCOLATES

Chocolates	Quantity (g)	Serving Size (g)	Protein (g) / 100 g	Fat (g) / 100 g	Fat Protein Calories (Kcal)	Fat Protein Unit (FPU)
5 Star	100	As Desired	1.80	16.00	151	2
Bourneville Rich Cocoa	100	80	4.70	34.60	330	3
Dairy Milk Chocolate	100	34	8.10	29.00	293	3
Dairy Milk Crackle	100	60	9.00	27.20	281	3
Dairy Milk Fruit and Nut	100	60	8.50	28.30	289	3
Dairy Milk Silk	100	As Desired	9.70	29.10	301	3
Dairy Milk Silk (Caramello)	100	60	5.10	24.40	240	2
Dairy Milk Silk (Roasted Almonds)	100	55	10.90	32.90	340	3
Dairy Milk Silk Oreo	100	22	6.20	34.90	339	3
Ferro Rocher	100	As Desired	8.20	42.70	417	4
Gems	100	As Desired	2.00	15.00	143	1
Kinder Joy	100	20	10.00	30.00	310	3
Lickables	100	20	6.00	32.00	312	3
Mentos	100	As Desired	0.08	0.41	4	0
Milky Bar	100	As Desired	4.70	15.30	157	2

(Contd.)

CHOCOLATES

Chocolates	Quantity (g)	Serving Size (g)	Protein (g) / 100 g	Fat (g) / 100 g	Fat Protein Calories (Kcal)	Fat Protein Unit (FPU)
Nestle Kit Kat	100	37	6.30	28.90	285	3
Nestle munch	100	11	5.90	22.60	227	2
Nutties	100	As Desired	5.70	26.40	260	3
Snickers	100	18	9.00	23.00	243	2
Temptations Rum Raisins	100	72	6.70	25.40	255	3

PROCESSED SNACKS

Processed Snacks	Quantity (g)	Serving Size (g)	Protein (g) / 100 g	Fat (g) / 100 g	Fat Protein Calories (Kcal)	Fat Protein Unit (FPU)
Corn Puffs	100	As Desired	6.65	11.16	127	1
Haldiram's Aloo Bhujia	100	As Desired	39.12	8.68	235	2
Haldiram's Bhujia Sev	100	As Desired	12.93	43.50	443	4
Haldiram's Moong Dal	100	As Desired	21.31	20.93	274	3
Kurkure	100	As Desired	6.30	35.70	347	3
Lays	100	As Desired	7.00	35.50	348	3

SPREADS

Spreads	Quantity (g)	Serving Size (g)	Protein (g) / 100 g	Fat (g) / 100 g	Fat Protein Calories (Kcal)	Fat Protein Unit (FPU)
Dr. Oetkar Eggless Sandwich Spread	100	As Desired	2.00	37.80	348	3
Fun Foods Peanut Butter Chocolate	100	As Desired	25.00	44.50	501	5
Fun Foods Veg Mayonnaise	100	As Desired	0.50	51.80	468	5
Hershey's Spread	100	As Desired	1.76	31.40	290	3
Nutella Hazelnut Spread	100	As Desired	2.00	12.00	116	1

READY TO MAKE FOODS

Ready to Make Foods	Quantity (g)	Serving Size (g)	Protein (g) / 100 g	Fat (g) / 100 g	Fat Protein Calories (Kcal)	Fat Protein Unit (FPU)
Aachi Lemon Rice Paste	100	As Desired	6.00	18.00	186	2
Aachi Tomato Garlic Rice Paste	100	As Desired	2.00	16.70	158	2
Act Ii Popcorn Classic Salted	100	As Desired	5.00	28.00	272	3
Betty Crocker Pan Cake Mix	100	22	5.50	7.70	91	1
Fresher Idiyappam	100	As Desired	4.10	0.00	16	0
ID Chapathi	100	39	7.70	5.58	81	1
ID Idly Batter	100	As Desired	5.50	1.60	36	0
Knorr Sweet Corn Mix	100	11	6.70	2.50	49	0
Knorr Tomato Soup Mix	100	13	5.40	5.70	73	1
Maggi Atta Masala Noodles	100	75	12.00	16.70	198	2
Maggi Masala Cup Noodles	100	70	8.30	19.20	206	2
Maggi Pasta (Cheese Macaroni)	100	70	11.50	3.50	78	1
Maggi Two Minutes Noodles	100	70	10.40	15.70	183	2
Manna Soya Nuggets	100	As Desired	52.00	1.00	217	2
Mccain Aloo Tikki	100	As Desired	2.46	5.55	60	1
Mccain Burger Patty	100	As Desired	3.72	8.86	95	1
Mccain Chilly Garlic Potato	100	As Desired	3.05	5.33	60	1
Mccain French Fries	100	As Desired	3.59	4.64	56	1
Mccain Mini Samosa	100	As Desired	8.34	12.16	143	1
Mccain Potato Cheese Shots	100	As Desired	8.09	11.30	134	1
Mccain Smileys	100	As Desired	2.97	7.73	81	1
Mccain Veg Fingers	100	As Desired	3.06	7.01	75	1

(Contd.)

READY TO MAKE FOODS

Ready to Make Foods	Quantity (g)	Serving Size (g)	Protein (g) / 100 g	Fat (g) / 100 g	Fat Protein Calories (Kcal)	Fat Protein Unit (FPU)
Mccain Veg Nuggets	100	As Desired	2.53	5.86	63	1
Mccain Wedges	100	As Desired	4.32	4.10	54	1
Modern Whole Wheat Parota	100	As Desired	9.30	12.10	146	1
Mother's Recipe Ginger Garlic Paste	100	16	3.00	0.00	12	0
Mtr Bajibonda	100	25	16.00	4.00	100	1
MTR Dal Makani	100	150	4.00	8.00	88	1
MTR Gulab Jamun	100	25	14.00	10.40	150	1
MTR Multigrain Dosa	100	45	12.00	5.00	93	1
Mtr Palak paneer	100	150	5.00	11.00	119	1
MTR Paneer Butter Masala	100	150	5.00	10.00	110	1
MTR Paneer Makani	100	150	5.00	15.00	155	2
Mtr Pongal	100	150	2.00	1.40	21	0
MTR Ragi Dosa	100	45	10.00	5.00	85	1
MTR Rava Dosai	100	45	9.00	2.50	59	1
MTR Rava Idli	100	40	4.00	3.20	45	0
MTR Rice Idli	100	40	13.00	2.50	75	1
MTR Sambar Rice	100	150	2.00	1.00	17	0
MTR Tomato Rice	100	125	1.00	3.00	31	0
Mtr Upma	100	70	10.00	11.00	139	1
Mtr Vada	100	As Desired	20.00	6.00	134	1
MTR Veg Pulao	100	125	3.00	6.50	71	1
MTR Vermicelli Kheer	100	As Desired	5.00	4.00	56	1
Pillsbury Eggless Cooker Cake	100	As Desired	8.10	6.70	93	1
Sunfeast Pasta Treat (Tomato)	100	70	11.50	3.70	79	1
Yipee Classic Masala Noodles	100	As Desired	20.00	12.00	188	2

READY TO EAT FOODS

Ready To Eat Foods	Quantity (g)	Serving Size (g)	Protein (g) / 100 g	Fat (g) / 100 g	Fat Protein Calories (Kcal)	Fat Protein Unit (FPU)
Haldirams Gulab jamun	100	26	6.58	12.36	138	1
Haldirams Rasagulla	100	26	8.52	1.12	44	0
Haldirams Son papdi	100	As Desired	7.66	30.04	301	3

READY TO MIX FOODS

Ready To Mix Foods	Quantity (g)	Serving Size (g)	Protein (g) / 100 g	Fat (g) / 100 g	Fat Protein Calories (Kcal)	Fat Protein Unit (FPU)
Bambino Gulab jamun	100	As Desired	17.00	12.70	182	2
Cadbury Hot chocolate	100	20	6.20	3.60	57	1
Cadbury Cocoa powder	100	As Desired	24.00	11.90	203	2
Hapima Fried rice mix	100	As Desired	21.50	1.70	101	1
Maggi Coconut powder	100	As Desired	6.50	50.20	478	5
Weikfield Caramel Pudding	100	As Desired	0.14	0.01	1	0
Weikfield Custard Powder	100	As Desired	1.30	0.40	9	0
Weikfield Falooda Mix	100	As Desired	2.41	0.45	14	0
Weikfield Jelly Crystals	100	As Desired	0.44	0.03	2	0

MISCELLANEOUS

Miscellaneous	Quantity (g)	Serving Size (g)	Protein (g) / 100 g	Fat (g) / 100 g	Fat Protein Calories (Kcal)	Fat Protein Unit (FPU)
Bindu Appalam	100	As Desired	25.02	0.26	102	1
Mother's Recipe Punjabi Masala Pappad	100	As Desired	17.00	3.00	95	1

Source: Nutritional Information from the Nutritional Label of the Packaged Food Product

Note:

- Nutrient values have been rounded off to the nearest number
- 1 Fat Protein Unit (FPU) = 100 Kcal
- All blank spaces in the table represent below the detectable limit
- FPU is calculated per 100gms of the Food Ingredients
- Nutritional information of processed and packaged foods have been retrieved from the Nutritional label of the packaged food product.
- Nutritional information of processed and packaged foods have been provided only for nutrient knowledge and not promotional purpose.
- Abbreviations: CHO - Carbohydrate, Cm - Centimeter, G - Gram, Kcal - Kilocalorie, Ml - Milliliter, No - Number, Tsp - Teaspoon, - - To be determined

FOOD INSULIN INDEX

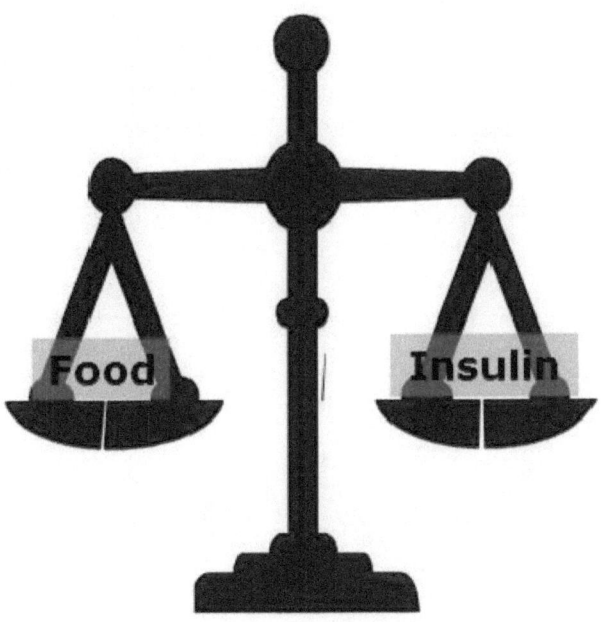

FOOD AND INSULIN

- Balance food and insulin
- Adapt insulin to suit meal
- Different regimens allow change in
- Meal plans
- Meal frequency

FOOD INSULIN INDEX

Food Insulin Index is testing iso energetic portions of single food (1000 KJ or 240 Kcals) in predicting insulin demand evoked by composite meals. Food Insulin Index is a better way to calculate insulin requirement compared to CHO counting or Glycemic Index.

An insulin index of foods may facilitate the day to day management of type I Diabetes. Although carbohydrate is the primary stimulus for insulin secretion, insulin tropic amino acids and bioactive peptides are also potent stimulators of insulin release. The lower Food Insulin Index will reduce the overall insulin demand or insulin requirement. The low insulinogenic calories are calculated by the formula.

$$\text{Insulinogenic calories} = \frac{(\text{CHO - fibre} + 0.54 \times \text{Protein}) \times 4\text{Kcals}}{\text{Total Calories}}$$

Examples of foods with low Food Insulin Index

FOOD	PROTEIN (g/MJ)	FAT (g/MJ)	CARBOHYDRATE (g/MJ)	Fiber (g/MJ)	INSULIN INDEX (%)
Butter	0	27	0	0	2
Peanut butter	9	20	7	5	11
Peanuts	10	20	5	2	15

Source: Optimizing nutrition, managing insulin (2015)

The Food Insulin Index may be useful in nutritional epidemiology because diets with high insulin demand have been hypothesized to increased risk of diabetes, obesity and cardiovascular disease. (Bao, Jong, Atkinson, Petocz& Brand-Miller, 2009).

References

1. Bao, J., Jong, V., Atkinson, F., Petocz, P., & Brand-Miller, J.C. (2009). Food Insulin Index: physiologic basis for predicting insulin demand evoked by composite meals, *American Journal of Clinical Nutrition, 90,* 986-992.
2. Holt, S.H., Mille, J.C., &Petocz, P.(1997). An insulin index of foods: the insulin demand generated by 1000- KJ portions of common foods, *American Journal Of Clinical Nutrition, 66*(5), 1264-1276.

FULLNESS FACTOR

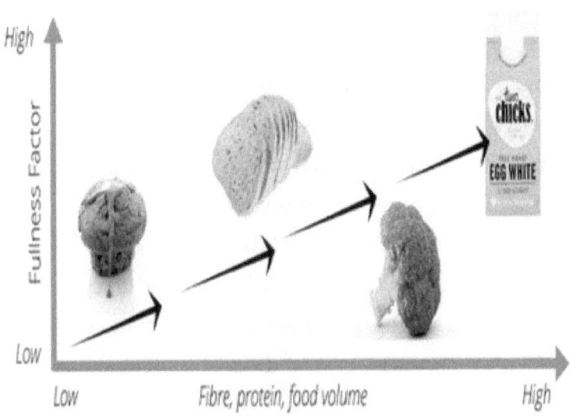

Your Diet Graph

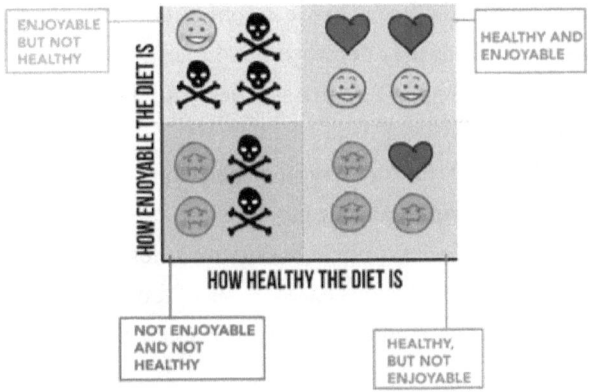

FULLNESS FACTOR

Satiation and satiety are two central concepts in the understanding of appetite control and both have to do with the inhibition of eating. "Satiation" refers to the end of *desire* to eat after a meal, and this can occur at any time after the onset of eating. "Satiety," on the other hand, is a physical feeling of fullness that allows us to stop eating for a while.

All calories are not treated by your body equally, the source of calories have more influence on satiety/ fullness. Ideally, satiety dwindles as nutrients diminish. Because when nutrients diminish, hunger returns. Satiety starts after the end of eating and prevents further eating before the return of hunger. This can be determined by a measured value called The Fullness Factor (FF).

Simple carbohydrates and starchy foods have a low effect on satiety and low Fullness Factors and are easy to be overeaten. On the other end, foods with high amounts of moisture, bulk, and/or protein have the greatest satiety and hence highest Fullness Factors. They include most vegetables, fruits, lean meats which fulfill the feeling of hunger. Fat has a similar effect on satiety as protein and fiber, which is why low-fat diets leave people hungry all the time. FF has well-defined advantages over the Glycemic Index. Hence FF needs to be taken into consideration while planning a low GI & low GL menu.

1. **FF can be easily determined for all foods**
    Standard nutrition facts label is required to determine the Fullness Factor, which means that the Fullness Factor is supported for all foods, and also for new recipes to use in conjunction with any diet plan.

2. **High-FF foods may decrease Total Energy Intake**
    Consuming high-FF foods satisfies your hunger with less total Calories.

3. **The Fullness Factor may also be helpful in planning weight losing/ gaining/ maintaining diets.**
    Individuals having trouble maintaining, losing or gaining weight can alter food selections based on FF of foods

Diets based on the Fullness Factor have some advantages over Low-Carb diets:

1. **FF-based diets stimulate the consumption of naturally healthy foods**

   Because many fruits, vegetables, and less processed foods have high Fullness Factors.

2. **FF-based diets offer a larger range of food selections**

   No foods are excluded from FF-based diets. These diets simply encourage selecting the foods that satiate rapidly without as many total Calories.

3. **FF-based diets can easily assist a vegetarian lifestyle**

   Lean meat cooked in healthy fats in moderation and served with fresh salads have a high FF. Even with vegetarian options, it is easy to create a high-FF diet. Sprouts with dry roasted healthy nuts accompanied with veggies /soups are optimal choices for a high-FF vegetarian diet.

Fat and fiber rich foods promote satiety. Fiber makes you satiated because it expands in your stomach. Fatty foods increase satiety because they take too long to digest. Fats and fiber both slow down the absorption of sugar. This leads to more stable blood sugars. Blood sugars play a role in determining hunger. These foods help shut off the hunger signal to your brain. Choice of foods based on satiating healthy food ingredients would help improve insulin sensitivity by achieving desired weight loss.

The Satiety Index evaluates satiety in comparison to white bread as the standard. Porridge is among the highest ranked foods by this measure.

Fullness Factors for Liquids

Most of the food items listed in the above table are solids; the Fullness Factor can also be calculated for liquids, including beverages. Majority of the liquid has above average Fullness Factors, due to their high moisture. Beverages do have a relatively high satiating effect that lasts for a brief period. However, low viscosity liquids (such as water, juice, or soft drinks) will be emptied from the stomach rapidly and leaves you hungry again in a relatively short time. Remember this, if you are using the Fullness Factor to select foods for weight loss.

FULLNESS FACTORS FOR COMMON FOODS

Food	FF
Bean sprouts	4.6
Watermelon	4.5
Grapefruit	4.0
Carrots	3.8
Oranges	3.5
Fish, broiled	3.4
Chicken breast, roasted	3.3
Apples	3.3
Sirloin steak, broiled	3.2
Oatmeal	3.0
Popcorn	2.9
Baked potato	2.5
Low-fat yogurt	2.5
Banana	2.5
Macaroni and cheese	2.5
Brown rice	2.3
Spaghetti	2.2
White rice	2.1
Pizza	2.1
Peanuts	2.0
Ice cream	1.8
White bread	1.8
Raisins	1.6
Snickers Bar	1.5
Honey	1.4
Sugar (sucrose)	1.3
Glucose	1.3
Potato chips	1.2
Butter	0.5

More filling per Calorie

Less filling per Calorie

Satiation occurs during an eating episode and brings it to an end

References

1. **Sweetness, Satiation, and Satiety**, France Bellisle Adam Drewnowski G. Harvey Anderson Margriet Westerterp- Plantenga Corby K. Martin*The Journal of Nutrition*, Volume 142, Issue 6, 1 June 2012, Pages 1149S–1154S, https://doi.org/10.3945/jn.111.149583, published: 09 May 2012
2. http://nutritiondata.self.com/topics/fullness-factor#ixzz5Jh SNTwpJ
3. http://nutritiondata.self.com/topics/glycemic-index#ixzz5JnQHeUgT

RENAL FOOD EXCHANGE LIST

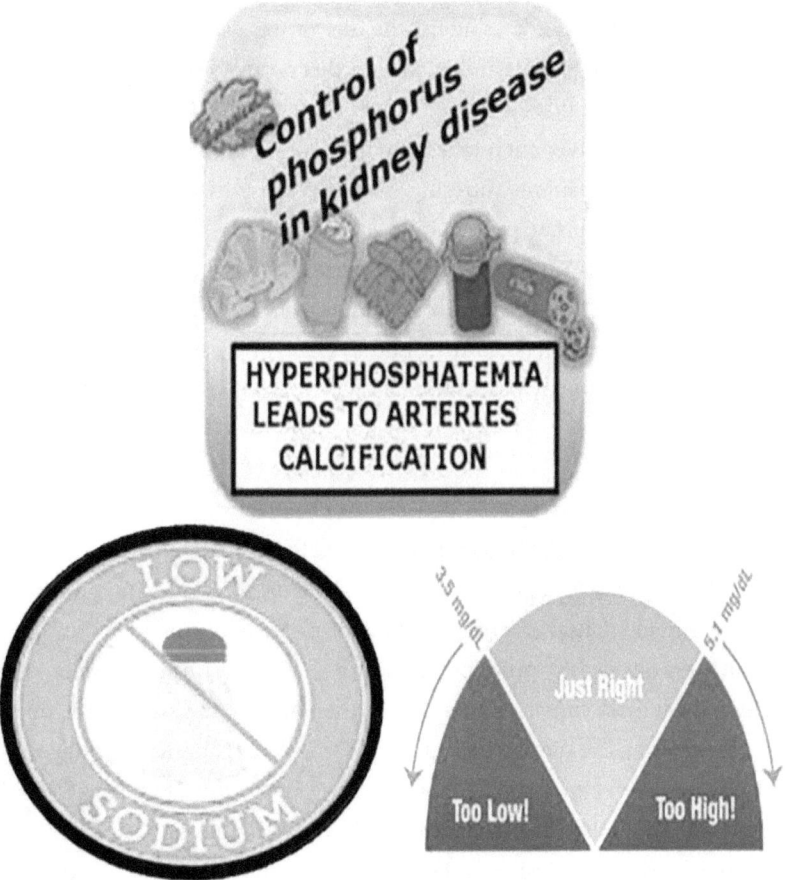

RENAL FOOD EXCHANGE LIST

The kidney Food Exchange list, also known as the Renal Food Exchange List, is a set of nutritional guidelines for people with kidney disease. The types of foods prescribed depend on the level of kidney failure the patient is experiencing, but generally, the diet involves controlling the amount of sodium, potassium, phosphorus, protein, and fluid that a person ingests.

Nutrition is essential for everyone but most important for the patients who suffer from metabolic and renal complication. Healthy kidneys help to regulate the amount of water, minerals, and electrolytes in the body. Improper functioning kidney needs to adjust the diet of the patients to maintain the delicate balance. If patients are on dialysis, diet needs to change even further. Menu planning includes -

- Optimal nutrient intake helps to improve nutritional status, quality of life in patients suffering from chronic kidney disease.
- An appropriate protein intake
- Limit the amount of salt (sodium), potassium and phosphorus based on their respective serum values.
- Limit fluid intake if urine output is less and patient suffering from swelling in any parts of the body.

Protein

A low protein diet (LPD) is generally advised for the patients with CKD, not on dialysis. Dietary protein is a source of nitrogen, phosphate, potassium and acid load. A higher protein intake of patients results in building up of nitrogenous waste products, hyperphosphatemia, hyperkalemia, and acidosis. All these impaired function further damage the kidney function.

Restricting the dietary proteins to 0.8 g/kg/d in patients with stage 3 to 5 CKD has been beneficial. Use of very low protein diets (0.3 g/kg/d) with ketoanalogues delays the initiation of dialysis. Patients on dialysis require 1.2 g/kg/d (hemodialysis) to 1.3 g/kg/d (peritoneal dialysis). Adequate energy should be provided for protein sparing action.

The below table shows the protein recommendation for various stages of Chronic Kidney Diseases.

Stages	Protein Recommendation
DPI of patients who are at risk of progression of CKD.	Should not exceed 1.3 g/kg/day
Stage 1 -3 in absence of malnutrition	0.75 g/kg/day
Stage 3 to 5 CKD	0.8 g/kg/day
CKD patients with or without diabetes mellitus and GFR < 30ml/min/1.73m2	0.8 g/kg/day
GFR< 25ml/min	Recommends 0.6 g/kg/day for patients
Patients on dialysis	1.2 g/kg/day (hemodialysis) to 1.3 g/kg/day (peritoneal dialysis).

Source: National Kidney Foundation, (2000)

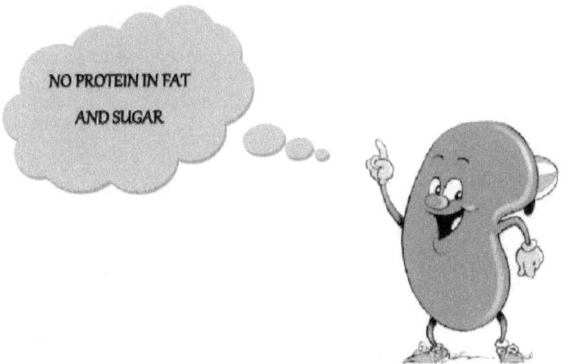

Potassium

Maintaining normal potassium levels is very important to prevent hypo and hyperkalemia which can be dangerous. When potassium levels raises in the blood, weakness of muscle, irregular heartbeat, and even death can occur. Limiting potassium in diet will help the patients with hyperkalemia to maintain the optimum levels of serum potassium.

Phosphorus

An important function of the kidney is to keep bones healthy by regulating the minerals calcium and phosphorus. The regulation of these minerals is affected when kidney function decreases. High blood phosphorus levels cause calcium to be leached out of the bone, leading to thinner and weaker bones. This condition is called osteodystrophy. Itching, bone pain, red eyes, and scaly skin can result from high phosphorus levels in the blood. Therapeutic strategies to control serum phosphorus levels include – dietary phosphorus restriction, decreased intestinal absorption with the use of phosphate binders and dialysis. To prevent the high levels of phosphorus in the diet, phosphorus intake should be reduced to lesser than 800-1000mgs/day in CKD stage 3 and 4 or when serum phosphorus levels >4.6mgdL or plasma PTH are elevated.

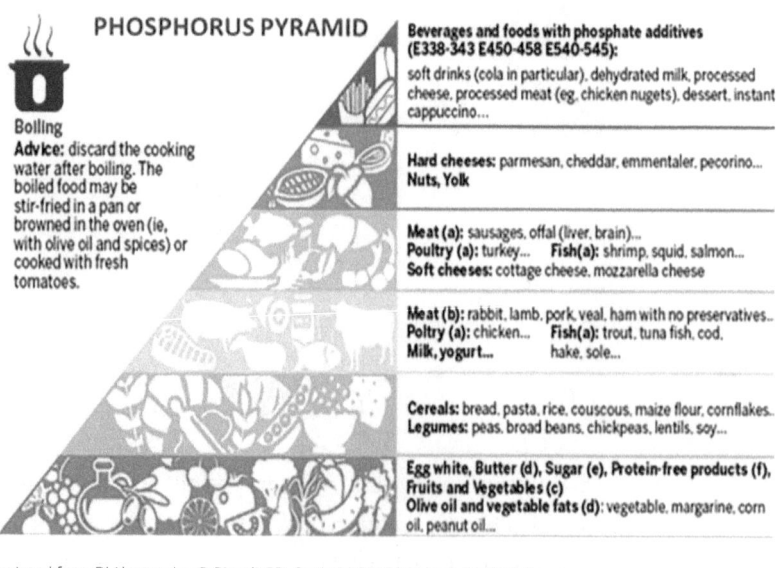

Reprinted from D' Alessandro C, Piccoli GB, Cupisti A.BMC Nephrol. 2015;16:9.

A one- size fits all sodium restriction is not possible. The CKD stage, amount of edema present, serum sodium level, blood pressure, ascites, overall nutritional status etc., and medications must be taken into consideration. There is consensus that high sodium intake is contraindicated for CKD.

Choosing sodium-free or low-sodium food products will help them maintain the normal serum level of sodium and fluid overload. Sodium restriction should be prescribed ranging from 1.5 – 2.3g/Na/day.

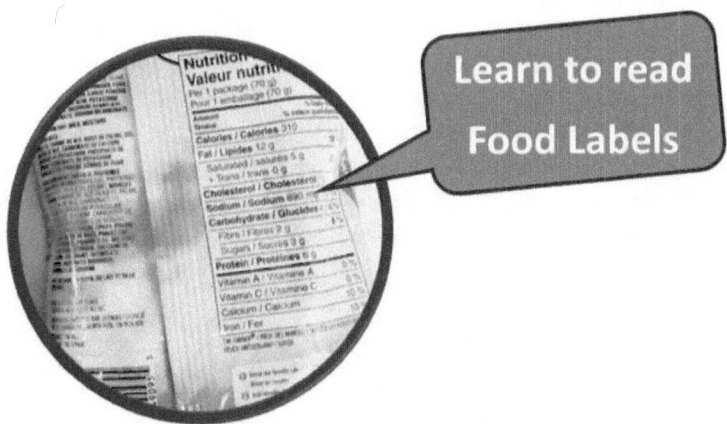

Fluid restrictions in patients with CKD are individualized based on excretory and obligatory losses.

Note:

Conversion	mmol	mg
Sodium	1	23
Potassium	1	39
Phosphorus	1	3

References

1. Arulraj, S. (Ed.). (2017). Cardio Diabetes Medicine, India, Bangalore: Micro Labs Limited.
2. Heerspink, H.J., Navis, G., & Ritz, E. (2012). Salt intake in kidney disease—a missed therapeutic opportunity? *Nephrology Dialysis Transplantation, 27*(9), 3435-3442.
3. KDIGO Kidney Disease: Improving Global Outcomes (KDIGO) CKD–MBD Work Group. (2009). KDIGO clinical practice guideline for the diagnosis, evaluation, prevention, and treatment of chronic kidney disease-mineral and bone disorder (CKD–MBD). *Kidney International Supplements, 113*, S1–S130.
4. Kidney Disease: Improving Global Outcomes (KDIGO) CKD Work Group. (2013). KDIGO 2012 Clinical Practice Guideline for the Evaluation and Management of Chronic Kidney Disease. *Kidney International Supplements, 3*, 1–150.
5. National Kidney Foundation. (2000). Clinical practice guidelines for nutrition in chronic renal failure, *American Journal of Kidney Disease, 35*, 1–140.
6. Nutrition and CKD. (n.d). Retrieved from http://renalmed.com/wp content/ uploads/2015/08/Nutrition-and-the-CKD-diet.pdf
7. Nutrition and CKD. (n.d). Retrieved from https://www.niddk.nih.gov/health-information/kidney-disease/chronic-kidney-disease-ckd/eating-nutrition/ nutrition-advanced-chronic-kidney-disease-adults

RENAL FOOD EXCHANGE LIST

Bajaj ,M., Kanagarajah, S., & Saloman, A

Tamil Nadu Government Multi Super Specialty Hospital, Chennai (2018)

FOOD INGREDIENT	Qty (g)/(ml)	Energy (kcal)	CHO (g)	Protein (g)	Fat (g)	Fibre (g)	Sodium (mg)	Potassium (mg)	Phosphorous (mg)
CEREAL RENAL EXCHANGE									
Cereals	25 g	85	17	3	1	2	1	47	42
Quinoa	25 g	85	17	3	1	2	1	119	53
MILLET RENAL EXCHANGE									
Millets	25 g	85	17	3	1	2	1	24	50
PULSE & WHOLE GRAM RENAL EXCHANGE									
Pulses	25 g	80	13	6	0.5	3	5	285	87
Whole grams	25 g	75	12	5	0	5	5	285	87
Soyabean	20 g	75	2	8	4	5	1	409	124
VEGETABLE RENAL EXCHANGE									
Group A (Green Leafy Vegetables)	100 g	35	3	4	1	5	24	413	58
Group B (Roots & Tubers)	100 g	50	10	1	0	3	26	388	47
Group C (Other Vegetables)	150 g	30	4	2	0	4	11	356	52

FOOD INGREDIENT	Qty (g)/(ml)	Energy (kcal)	CHO (g)	Protein (g)	Fat (g)	Fibre (g)	Sodium (mg)	Potassium (mg)	Phosphorous (mg)
Onion	100g	52	11	2	1	1	5	166	36
Fruit Renal Exchange	90 g	40	8	1	0	3	3	169	17
Fruits with Potassium <100 mg	90 g	40	8	1	0	3	3	94	8
Fruits with Potassium (100-200)mg	100 g	40	8	1	0	3	3	141	14
Fruits with Potassium >200mg	100 g	40	8	1	0	3	2	245	25
MILK & MILK PRODUCTS									
Cow's Milk	100 ml	73	5	3.3	4.5	0	25	115	97
Skimmed milk*	100 ml	29	4	2.5	0	0	0	NA	9
EGG RENAL EXCHANGE									
Egg, country ,hen whole, raw	50 g	84	0	6.6	6.5	0	79	59	99
Egg, poultry , whole, raw	50 g	67	0	6.6	4.5	0	62	69	93
ANIMAL MEAT & MARINE RENAL EXCHANGE									
Animal Meat	75g	75	0	13	2	0	29	253	146
Marine Fish & Shellfish	75g	75	0	13	2	0	57	265	186
Prawns, big	75g	75	0	13	2	0	637	202	178
SUGARS									
Sago	10 g	40	10	0	0	0	NA	NA	NA

FOOD INGREDIENT	Qty (g)/(ml)	Energy (kcal)	CHO (g)	Protein (g)	Fat (g)	Fibre (g)	Sodium (mg)	Potassium (mg)	Phosphorous (mg)
Jaggery	10 g	40	10	0	0	0	3	49	8
Sugar	10 g	40	10	0	0	0	0	0	NA
FATS & NUTS RENAL EXCHANGE									
Nuts	15 g	85	2	3	7	1.5	1	94	59
Fat	10 g	90	0	0	10	0	0	0	0

Note:

- The meal planning food exchange list depicts the average value of the macronutrients of the food items in each exchange list described in the following individual exchange tables
- Nutrient values have been rounded off to the nearest number
- Abbreviation: Qty - Quantity, g - gram, ml - millilitre, Kcal - kilocalorie, CHO – Carbohydrate, NA-Not Available

References

1. Longvah, T., Ananthan, R., Bhaskarachary, K.., &Venkaiah, K. (2017). Indian Food Composition Tables, India, Hyderabad: National Institute of Nutrition.

2. Gopalan, C., Sastri, B.V.R, & Balasubramanian, S. C. (1989). Nutritive Value of Indian Foods (Rev.ed.). India, Hyderabad: National Institute of Nutrition.

RENAL FOOD EXCHANGE LIST

Bajaj , M., Kanagarajah,S., & Saloman, A
Tamil Nadu Government Multi Super Specialty Hospital, Chennai (2018)

	Raw Weight (g)	Sodium (mg)	Potassium (mg)	Phosphorus (mg)
Cereal				
Chapati, whole wheat flour	25	1	78	79
Rice flakes (dry)	25	1	37	49
Rice, Parboiled milled	25	1	36	35
Rice, raw milled	25	1	27	24
Wheat flour, refined	25	0	37	28
Wheat, Semolina (dry)	25	1	71	30
Wheat, Vermicelli (dry)	25	1	41	49
CEREAL RENAL EXCHANGE *	25	1	47	42
Quinoa	25	1	119	53
Millet				
Bajra	25	1	91	72
Jowar	25	1	82	69
Ragi	25	1	111	53
Samai	25	1	26	33
Varagu	25	1	24	25
MILLET RENAL EXCHANGE*	25	1	67	50
Pulse & Whole Gram				
Bengal gram, dhal	25	5	239	81
Bengal gram, whole	25	7	233	67
Black gram, dhal	25	5	289	94
Black gram, whole	25	7	273	86

	Raw Weight (g)	Sodium (mg)	Potassium (mg)	Phosphorus (mg)
Cow pea, white	25	3	310	95
Green gram, dhal	25	3	317	104
Green gram, whole	25	3	294	88
Horse gram, whole	25	3	266	75
Peas dry	25	6	230	84
Rajma,red	25	3	331	102
Red gram, dhal	25	5	348	82
PULSE & WHOLE GRAM RENAL EXCHANGE*	25	5	285	87
SOYABEAN,WHITE	20	1	409	124
VEGETABLE EXCHANGE LIST				
Vegetable A (Green Leafy Vegetables)				
Agathi leaves	100	18	674	53
Amaranth leaves, green	100	16	572	73
Cabbage, green	100	15	233	30
Cauliflower leaves	100	24	374	63
Drumstick leaves	100	9	397	109
Fenugreek leaves	100	47	226	53
Lettuce	100	18	279	44
Mustard leaves	100	19	403	72
Ponangani	100	39	457	58
Radish leaves	100	17	304	50
Spinach	100	43	625	33
GREEN LEAFY VEGETABLES RENAL EXCHANGE*	100	24	413	58
Group B Vegetables (Roots & Tubers)				
Beetroot	100	69	306	36
Carrot, orange	100	52	273	43

	Raw Weight (g)	Sodium (mg)	Potassium (mg)	Phosphorus (mg)
Colocasia	100	5	514	81
Potato, brown skin, big	100	4	541	43
Sweet potato, Pink skin	100	29	329	38
Tapioca	100	11	255	43
Yam, elephant	100	14	501	43
ROOTS & TUBERS RENAL EXCHANGE*	**100**	**26**	**388**	**47**
Group C Vegetables (Other Vegetables)				
Ash gourd#	150	2	558	44
Beans scarlet, tender#	150	2	246	93
Bitter gourd, jagged, teethridges, elongate	150	20	489	68
Bottle gourd, elongate, pale green#	150	2	186	24
Brinjal all varieties#	150	2	371	50
Cauliflower	150	46	494	71
Cucumber, green elongate#	150	10	275	43
Ladies finger	150	11	395	86
Plantain flower^	150	11	732	71
Ridge gourd	150	7	177	50
Snake gourd,long,pale green	150	11	150	35
Tomato, Green	150	20	338	34
Tomato, red ripe local	150	15	306	28
Zucchini, green	150	1	267	32
OTHER VEGETABLES RENAL EXCHANGE	**150**	**11**	**356**	**52**
# Sodium is 2, ^Potassium is 732				
Onion, big	100	6	171	32
Onion, small	100	4	160	40
ONION RENAL EXCHANGE*	**100**	**5**	**166**	**36**

	Raw Weight (g)	Sodium (mg)	Potassium (mg)	Phosphorus (mg)
Fruit				
Jambufruit , ripe	90	3	93	9
Pear	90	2	95	6
Apple,big	90	1	104	9
Grapes, green round seeded	90	2	149	18
Mango, ripe, banganapalli	90	1	130	10
Musk melon , orange flesh	90	13	185	16
Orange, pulp	90	1	148	12
Papaya, ripe	90	6	156	16
Pineapple	90	1	129	13
Plum	90	1	146	13
Strawberry	90	1	126	23
Lime Sweet, pulp	90	1	164	19
Watermelon, dark green	90	2	112	10
Custard apple	90	3	250	37
Dates, processed	90	1	260	31
Gooseberry	90	1	201	20
Guava, white flesh	90	3	255	22
Jackfruit, ripe	90	2	251	21
Sapota	90	4	252	20
FRUIT RENAL EXCHANGE*	90	3	169	17
Condiments & Spices				
Asafoetida	10	2	25	7
Cardamom, green	10	2	126	13
Chillies, green all varieties	10	0	34	5
Coriander leaves	10	4	55	7
Curry leaves	10	2	58	8

	Raw Weight (g)	Sodium (mg)	Potassium (mg)	Phosphorus (mg)
Fenugreek seed	10	4	89	44
Garlic, big clove	10	1	43	12
Ginger, fresh	10	1	41	4
Mint leaves	10	2	54	7
Poppy seeds	10	3	65	80
Cloves	10	18	143	8
Coriander seed	10	3	147	29
Cumin seed	10	13	189	38
Omum	10	3	169	33
Pepper, black	10	2	149	14
Chillies, red	10	2	225	28
Turmeric powder	10	2	237	28
Nuts & Oilseeds				
Cashew	15	1	95	75
Coconut, Kernel, Fresh	15	1	37	10
Walnut	15	0	68	60
Almond	15	0	105	67
Groundnut	15	2	102	59
Pistachio nut	15	1	158	81
NUTS AND OIL SEEDS RENAL EXCHANGE*	15	1	94	59
Sugars				
Honey**	10	NA	NA	2
Jaggery	10	3	49	8
Sago	10	NA	NA	NA
Sugar**	10	0	0	NA
SUGAR RENAL EXCHANGE	10	3	49	5

Source: IFCT (2017) & NIN (1989)**

	Raw Weight (g/ml)	Sodium (mg)	Potassium (mg)	Phosphorus (mg)
Milk & Milk Products				
Paneer	100 g	18	64	330
Curd**	100 g	32	130	93
Milk, whole, Buffalo	100 ml	30	109	87
Milk, whole, Cow	100 ml	25	115	97
Buttermilk (cow's milk)**	100 ml	0	NA	30
Skimmed milk**	100 ml	0	NA	90
Skimmed milk powder**	100 g	0	NA	1000

Source: IFCT (2017) & NIN (1989)**

	Egg & Animal Meat			
Beef, chops	75	24	287	157
Chicken, poultry, breast, skinless	75	28	221	134
Goat, chops	75	34	251	146
COUNTRY, ANIMAL MEAT RENAL EXCHANGE*	**75**	**29**	**253**	**146**
Egg, poultry, whole raw	50	79	59	99
Egg, poultry , whole, raw	50	62	69	93
MARINE (FISH & SHELLFISH)				
Marine Fish				
Anchovy (Nethili)	75	159	203	185
Paarai (Jack fish)	75	34	288	213
Pomfret, black	75	52	221	146
Salmon fish	75	15	259	158
Vanjaram (Seer fish)	75	26	355	227
MARINE FISH RENAL EXCHANGE*	**75**	**57**	**265**	**186**
Marine Shellfish				
Prawns , big	75	637	202	178

Note:

- The meal planning food exchange list depicts the average value of the macronutrients of the food items in each exchange list described in the following individual exchange tables
- Nutrient values have been rounded off to the nearest number
- Abbreviation: Qty - Quantity, g - gram, ml - millilitre, Kcal - kilocalorie, CHO - Carbohydrate
- Average*
- LOW POTASSIUM   : Potassium < 100mg/exchange
- MEDIUM POTASSIUM : Potassium (100–200)mg/exchange
- HIGH POTASSIUM   : Potassium > 200mg/exchange

References

1. Longvah, T., Ananthan, R., Bhaskarachary, K.., &Venkaiah, K. (2017). Indian Food Composition Tables, India, Hyderabad: National Institute of Nutrition.
2. Gopalan, C., Sastri, B.V.R., & Balasubramanian, S. C. (1989). Nutritive Value of Indian Foods (Rev.ed.). India, Hyderabad: National Institute of Nutrition

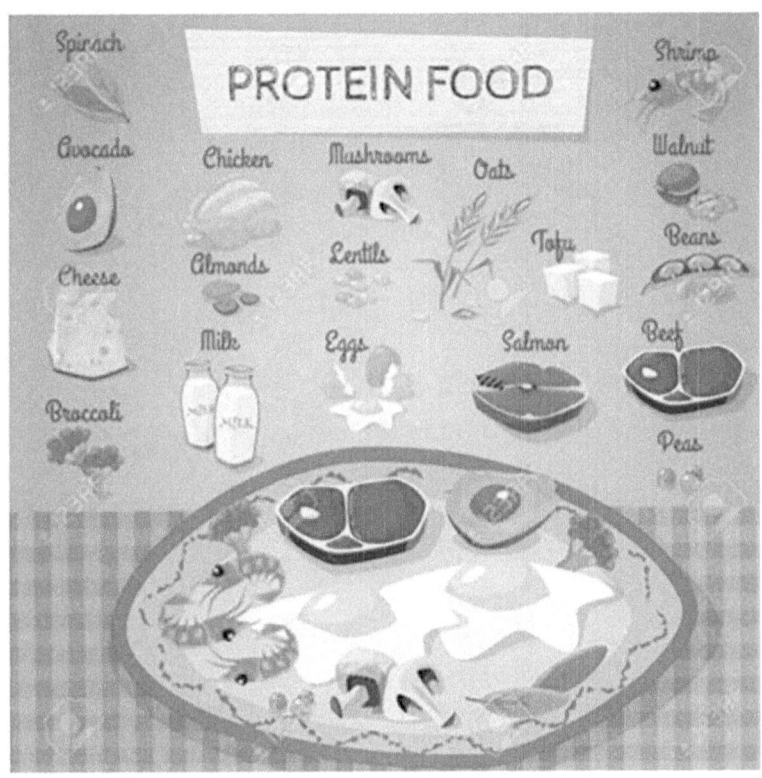

PROTEIN CONTENT IN VARIOUS FOOD CATEGORIES

Bajaj, M., Begam, S., & Fahmitha, N.

Tamilnadu Government Multi Super Speciality Hospital, Chennai (2018)

FOOD ITEMS

A	Protein in Cereal Exchange List	Raw Weight (g)	Protein (g)
	Processed Cereals		
	Kellogg's Cornflakes	44	3
	Modern Sweet Bread(1 slice -10cm width, Thickness- 1cm)	25	3
	Quaker Oats	26	3
	Unprocessed Cereals		
	Barley	27	3
	Chapati, whole wheat flour	28	3
	Dosa flour (dry)	28	3
	Idly (dry)	28	3
	Quinoa	23	3
	Rice flakes (dry)	40	3
	Rice, Parboiled milled	39	3
	Rice, raw milled	39	3
	Wheat flour, refined	29	3
	Wheat, Wheat, Semolina (dry)	27	3
	Wheat, Vermicelli (dry)	31	3
B	**Protein In Millet Exchange List**	Raw Weight (g)	Protein (g)
	Bajra	64	7
	Jowar	70	7
	Ragi	98	7
	Samai	69	7
	Varagu	78	7
C	**Protein In Pulse Exchange List**	Raw Weight (g)	Protein (g)
	Bengal gram, dal	33	7
	Bengal gram, whole	37	7
	Black gram, dal	30	7
	Black gram, whole	32	7

(Contd.)

Cowpea, white	33	7
Green gram, dal	29	7
Green gram, whole	31	7
Horse gram, whole	32	7
Peas dry	34	7
Rajma, red	35	7
Red gram, dal	32	7
Soyabean, white	19	7

D	Protein In Vegetable Exchange List	Raw Weight (g)	Protein (g)
	Group A (Green Leafy Vegetables)		
	Agathi	17	2
	Amaranth, green	41	2
	Cabbage leaves, green	98	2
	Cauliflower leaves	34	2
	Drumstick	21	2
	Fenugreek	36	2
	Lettuce	87	2
	Mustard leaves	38	2
	Ponnanganni	25	2
	Radish leaves	60	2
	Spinach leaves	62	2
	Group B (Roots and Tubers)		
	Beetroot	69	2
	Carrot, Orange	141	2
	Colocasia	41	2
	Potato, brown skin big	87	2
	Sweet potato, Pink skin	106	2
	Tapioca	131	2
	Yam, elephant	53	2

Group C (Other Vegetables)		
Ash gourd	169	2
Beans scarlet, tender	47	2
Bitter gourd, jagged, teethridges, elongate	97	2
Bottle gourd, elongate, pale green	252	2
Brinjal all varieties	91	2
Cauliflower	62	2
Cucumber, green elongate	189	2
Ladies finger	65	2
Plantain flower	91	2
Ridge gourd	147	2
Snake gourd, long, pale green	136	2
Tomato (Green)	119	2
Tomato (red ripe)	148	2
Zucchini	121	2

E	Protein in Fruit Exchange List	Raw Weight (g)	Protein (g)
	Apple, big	173	0.5
	Banana, poovam	34	0.5
	Custard apple	31	0.5
	Dates, processed	44	0.5
	Gooseberry	160	0.5
	Grapes, green round seeded	66	0.5
	Guava, white flesh	35	0.5
	Jackfruit, ripe	18	0.5
	Jambu fruit, ripe	61	0.5
	Mango, ripe, banganapalli	93	0.5
	Muskmelon, orange flesh	120	0.5
	Orange, pulp	72	0.5
	Papaya, ripe	119	0.5

(Contd.)

	Pear	129	0.5
	Pineapple	96	0.5
	Plum	79	0.5
	Sapota	54	0.5
	Strawberry	52	0.5
	Sweet lime, pulp	66	0.5
	Tamarind, pulp	17	0.5
	Watermelon, dark green	83	0.5
F	**Protein in Milk Exchange List**	**Raw Weight (g)**	**Protein (g)**
	Buttermilk (cow's milk)*	500 ml	4
	Curd*	129 g	4
	Milk, whole, Buffalo	109 ml	4
	Milk, whole, Cow	123 ml	4
	Paneer	21 g	4
	Skimmed milk powder*	11 g	4
	Skimmed milk*	160 ml	4
G	**Protein in Meat Exchange List**	**Raw Weight (g)**	**Protein (g)**
	Beef chops	36	7
	Chicken, poultry, breast, skinless	32	7
	Egg, poultry, whole, raw	53	7
	Goat, chops	34	7
H	**Protein in Marine Exchange List**	**Raw Weight (g)**	**Protein (g)**
	Anchovy (Nethili)	35	7
	Paarai (Jackfish)	32	7
	Pomfret, black	37	7
	Prawns, big	36	7
	Salmon fish	33	7
	Vanjaram (Seer fish)	31	7

I	Protein in Condiments and Spices	Raw Weight (g)	Protein (g)
	Asafoetida	110	7
	Cardamom, green	86	7
	Chilies, green	297	7
	Chilies, red	55	7
	Cloves	119	7
	Coriander leaves	199	7
	Coriander seed	66	7
	Cumin seed	50	7
	Curry leaves	94	7
	Fenugreek seed	28	7
	Garlic, big clove	101	7
	Ginger, fresh	315	7
	Mint leaves	150	7
	Omum	44	7
	Onion, big	467	7
	Onion, small	385	7
	Pepper, black	69	7
	Poppy seeds	34	7
	Turmeric powder	91	7
J	Protein in Nuts Exchange	Raw Weight (g)	Protein (g)
	Almond	38	7
	Cashew	32	7
	Coconut, kernel, fresh	184	7
	Groundnut	30	7
	Mustard seed	36	7
	Pistachios nut	30	7
	Walnut	47	7

(Contd.)

K	Protein in Sugars	Raw Weight (g)	Protein (g)
	Sago*	3500	0
	Honey*	2333	0
	Jaggery	378	0

RETRIEVED FROM: IFCT (2017), NIN (1989)*

Note:

- Since the protein content for fats & oils are below detectable amounts, the protein content in fat exchange is considered as zero.
- Nutrient values have been rounded off to the nearest number.
- Abbreviation : gm- gram, ml –milli litre, no-number

References

1. Longvah, T., Ananthan, R., Bhaskarachary, K., &Venkaiah, K. (2017). *Indian Food Composition Tables*, India, Hyderabad: National Institute of Nutrition.
2. * Gopalan, C., Sastri, B .V. R., & Balasubramanian, S. C. (1989). *Nutritive Value of Indian Foods (Rev.ed.)*. India, Hyderabad: National Institute of Nutrition.
3. ** Susan, E., Gebhardt., Robin, G., & Thomas. (2002). *Nutritive Value of Foods*, U.S Department of Agriculture.

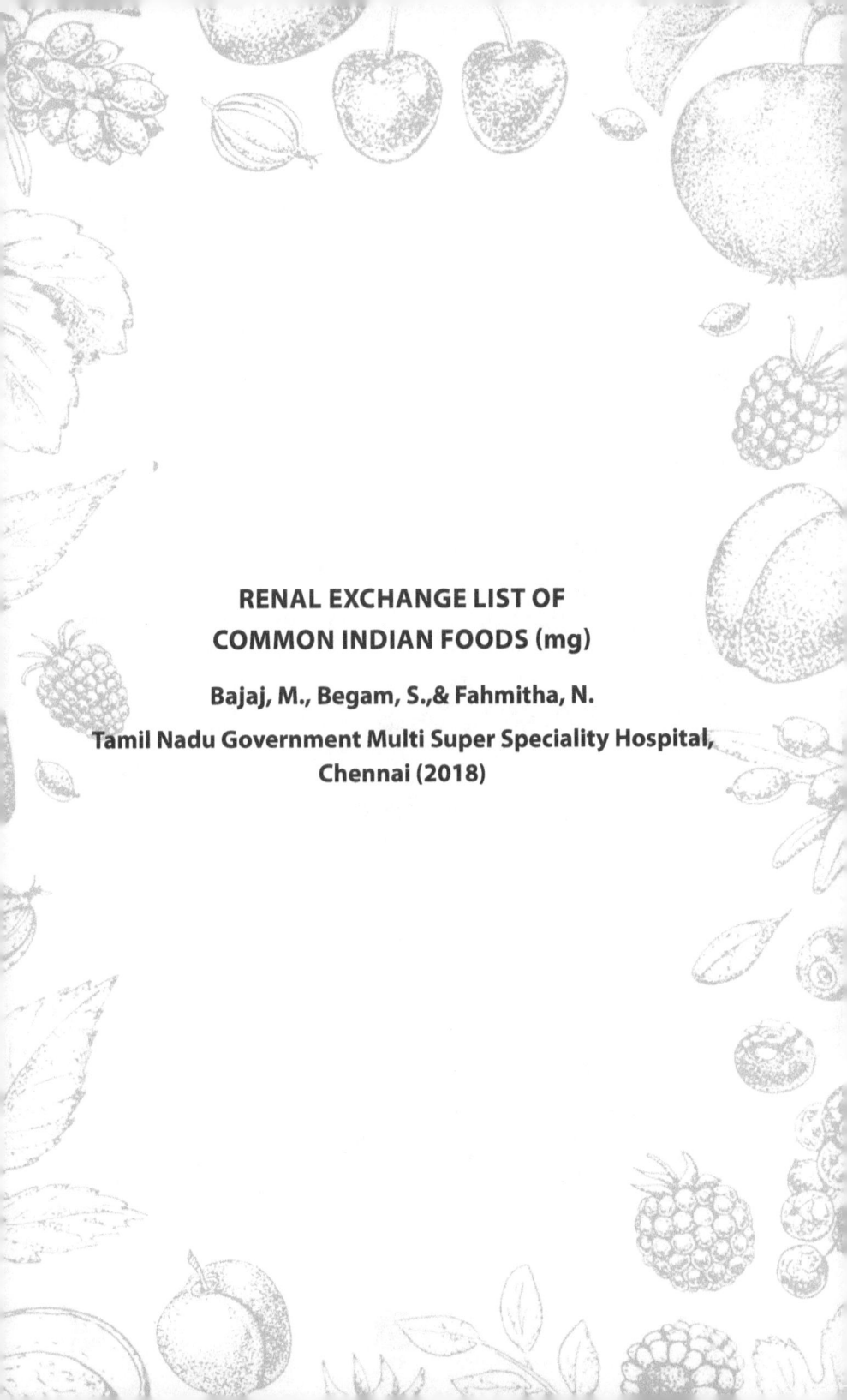

RENAL EXCHANGE LIST OF COMMON INDIAN FOODS (mg)

Bajaj, M., Begam, S.,& Fahmitha, N.

Tamil Nadu Government Multi Super Speciality Hospital, Chennai (2018)

Food Ingredient	Raw Weight (g)	Sodium (mg)	Potassium (mg)	Phosphorus (mg)
Cereal				
Barley	100	8	268	178
Dosa flour (dry)	100	788	332	181
Idly flour (dry)	100	788	332	181
Quinoa	100	5	474	212
Rice flakes (dry)	100	3	148	195
Rice, Parboiled milled	100	3	142	140
Rice, raw milled	100	2	108	96
Wheat flour, refined	100	2	148	110
Wheat, Semolina (dry)	100	2	284	119
Wheat, Vermicelli (dry)	100	3	163	99
Whole wheat flour	100	2	311	315
Millet				
Bajra	100	4	365	289
Jowar	100	5	328	274
Ragi	100	5	443	210
Samai	100	5	105	130
Varagu	100	3	94	101
Pulse				
Bengal gram, dhal	100	21	957	325
Bengal gram, whole	100	27	935	267
Black gram, dhal	100	19	1157	375
Black gram, whole	100	27	1093	345
Cow pea, white	100	13	1243	378

Food Ingredient	Raw Weight (g)	Sodium (mg)	Potassium (mg)	Phosphorus (mg)
Green gram, dhal	100	10	1268	416
Green gram, whole	100	12	1177	353
Horse gram, whole	100	12	1065	298
Peas dry	100	23	922	334
Rajmah,red	100	10	1324	409
Red gram, dhal	100	18	1395	328
Soyabean,white	100	3	1634	494
Group A Vegetables (Green Leafy Vegetables)				
Agathi leaves	100	18	674	53
Amaranth leaves, green	100	16	572	73
Cabbage, green	100	14	233	30
Cauliflower leaves	100	24	374	63
Drumstick leaves	100	10	397	109
Fenugreek leaves	100	47	226	53
Lettuce	100	18	279	44
Mustard leaves	100	19	403	72
Ponnaganni	100	39	457	58
Radish leaves	100	17	304	50
Spinach	100	43	625	33
Group B Vegetables (Roots & Tubers)				
Beetroot	100	69	306	36
Carrot, orange	100	52	273	43
Colocasia	100	5	514	81
Potato, brown skin, big	100	4	541	43

(Contd.)

Food Ingredient	Raw Weight (g)	Sodium (mg)	Potassium (mg)	Phosphorus (mg)
Sweet potato, Pink skin	100	29	329	38
Tapioca	100	11	255	43
Yam, elephant	100	14	501	43
Group C (Other Vegetables)				
Ash gourd	100	1	372	29
Beans scarlet, tender	100	1	164	62
Bitter gourd, jagged, teethridges, elongate	100	13	326	45
Bottle gourd, elongate, pale green	100	1	124	16
Brinjal all varieties	100	4	247	33
Cauliflower	100	31	329	47
Cucumber, green elongate	100	6	183	28
Ladies finger	100	7	263	57
Plantain flower	100	8	488	47
Ridge gourd	100	5	118	33
Snake gourd,long,pale green	100	7	100	23
Tomato, Green	100	13	225	23
Tomato, red ripe local	100	10	204	19
Zucchini, green	100	0	178	21
Fruit				
Apple, big	100	1	116	10
Banana, ripe, poovam	100	1	335	34
Custard apple	100	3	278	41

Food Ingredient	Raw Weight (g)	Sodium (mg)	Potassium (mg)	Phosphorus (mg)
Dates, processed	100	2	289	34
Gooseberry	100	1	223	22
Grapes, green round seeded	100	2	166	20
Guava, white flesh	100	3	283	24
Jackfruit, ripe	100	2	279	23
Jambufruit, ripe	100	3	103	10
Mango, ripe, banganapalli	100	1	144	11
Musk melon , orange flesh	100	15	206	17
Orange, pulp	100	1	164	13
Papaya, ripe	100	7	173	18
Pear	100	2	106	7
Pineapple	100	1	143	14
Plum	100	2	162	14
Sapota	100	5	280	22
Strawberry	100	1	140	26
Sweet lime, pulp	100	1	182	21
Tamarind, pulp	100	25	836	113
Watermelon, dark green	100	2	124	11
Milk & Milk Products				
Buttermilk (cow's milk)*	100 ml	0	NA	30
Curd*	100 g	32	130	93
Milk, whole, Buffalo	100 ml	30	109	87
Milk, whole, Cow	100 ml	25	115	97
Paneer	100 g	18	64	330

(Contd.)

Food Ingredient	Raw Weight (g)	Sodium (mg)	Potassium (mg)	Phosphorus (mg)
Skimmed milk powder*	100 g	0	NA	1000
Skimmed milk*	100 ml	0	NA	90
Egg & Animal Meat				
Beef, chops	100	32	383	209
Chicken, poultry, breast, skinless	100	37	295	178
Egg, poultry, whole raw	100	123	138	185
Goat, chops	100	46	334	195
Marine Fish				
Anchovy (Nethili)	100	212	270	246
Paarai (Jack fish)	100	45	384	284
Pomfret, black	100	69	295	195
Prawns , big	100	849	269	237
Salmon fish	100	20	345	211
Vanjaram (Seer fish)	100	35	473	302
Condiments & Spices				
Asafoetida	100	16	245	69
Cardamom, green	100	16	1262	132
Chillies, green all varieties	100	3	341	51
Chillies, red	100	19	2245	280
Cloves	100	183	1434	83
Coriander leaves	100	37	546	65
Coriander seed	100	34	1473	293
Cumin seed	100	125	1886	382
Curry leaves	100	19	584	83

Food Ingredient	Raw Weight (g)	Sodium (mg)	Potassium (mg)	Phosphorus (mg)
Fenugreek seed	100	40	891	435
Garlic, big clove	100	9	430	119
Ginger,fresh	100	10	407	44
Mint leaves	100	17	539	65
Omum	100	29	1692	329
Onion, big	100	6	171	32
Onion, small	100	4	160	40
Pepper, black	100	24	1487	144
Poppy seeds	100	25	646	804
Turmeric powder	100	24	2374	276
Nuts & Oilseeds				
Almond	100	2	699	446
Cashew	100	9	635	500
Coconut, Kernel, Fresh	100	8	246	68
Groundnut	100	12	679	391
Mustard seed	100	4	694	715
Pistachio nut	100	7	1053	537
Walnut	100	1	457	400
Sugars				
Honey*	100	NA	NA	18
Jaggery	100	25	488	76
Sago*	100	NA	NA	NA
Sugar**	100	1	2	NA

Note:

- Retrieved from IFCT (2017), NIN (1989)*& USDA (2002)**
- Abbreviations: NA - Not Available, Zero - "0" Below detectable limit

(Contd.)

RENAL EXCHANGE LIST OF PROCESSED FOOD

Bajaj, M., Begam, S., & Fahmitha, N.

Tamil Nadu Government Multi Super Speciality Hospital, Chennai (2018)

Processed Foods	Raw Weight (g)	Sodium (mg)	Potassium (mg)	Phosphorus (mg)
PROCESSED CEREALS				
Modern Sweet Bread	100	NA	NA	NA
Quaker Oats	100	4	NA	NA
Kellogg's Cornflakes	100	1	NA	NA
Tetrapack Juices				
Tropicana - Orange	100	34	82	NA
Real – Pomegranate	100	40	50	NA
Carbonated Beverages				
Pepsi	100	11	NA	NA
Mount Dew	100	16	NA	NA
Pickles				
777 Mango Pickle	100	4650	NA	NA
Instant Soup				
Knorr Mixed Vegetable Soup	100	3712	NA	NA
Chings Sweet Corn Veg Soup	100	5725	NA	NA
Chocolate				
Diary Milk	100	152	NA	NA
Noodles				
Maggi Noodles	100	1286	NA	NA
Knorr Mast Masala Noodles	100	1904	NA	NA
Appalam				
BinduAppalam	100	1	NA	NA
Popcorn				
Act II Popcorn (Golden Sizzle)	100	2	NA	NA
American Garden - Cheese Popcorn	100	970	NA	NA

Processed Foods	Raw Weight (g)	Sodium (mg)	Potassium (mg)	Phosphorus (mg)
Biscuit				
Cadbury Original Oreo Sandwich Biscuit	100	498	NA	NA
Ketchup				
Kissan Ketchup	100	907	NA	NA
Jam				
Kissan Jam	100	20	NA	NA
Sauce				
Jerrys Chilli Sauce	100	4692	189	NA
Milk Products				
Britannia Cheese Cubes	100	1439	NA	584
Nestle Milk Maid	100	140	NA	NA
Amul Butter	100	836	NA	NA
Health Drinks				
Horlicks	100	400	450	280
Ovaltin	100	90	NA	NA
Squash and Instant Drink Mix				
Kissan Orange Squash	100	60	37	NA
Tang Orange Instant Drink Mix	100	29	NA	NA
Namkeen				
Kurkure Aloo Bhujia	100	920	NA	NA
HaldiramsBhujiaSev	100	788	NA	NA
Renal Supplements (Oral Nutrition / Enteral)				
Essential Renal	100	26	110	175
Fresubin HP	100	140	235	140
Fresubin LP	100	111	133	192

(Contd.)

Processed Foods	Raw Weight (g)	Sodium (mg)	Potassium (mg)	Phosphorus (mg)
Kabipro #	100	230	685	390
Nepro HP	100	149	282	191
Nepro LP	100	171	312	195
Pentasure DLS	100	140	235	143
Pentasure Renal	100	113	137	191
Proseventy	100	775	292	700
Real HP	100	280	480	200
Resource Dialysis	100	270	460	170
Resource Renal	100	250	414	145

Note:

- Source :Retrieved From: Nutritional information from the Nutritional label of the packaged food product
- Nutrient values have been rounded off to the nearest number
- Since the sodium, potassium, phosphorus content for fats & oils are below detectable amounts, the sodium, potassium, phosphorus content for this exchanges expressed as zero.
- Potassium is in micrograms
- Abbreviation: NA – Not available.

References

1. Longvah, T., Ananthan, R., Bhaskarachary, K., &Venkaiah, K. (2017). Indian Food Composition Tables, India, Hyderabad: National Institute of Nutrition.
2. * Gopalan, C., Sastri, B.V. R.,& Balasubramanian, S. C. (1989). Nutritive Value of Indian Foods (Rev.ed.). India, Hyderabad: National Institute of Nutrition.
3. ** Susan, E., Gebhardt., Robin, G., &Thomas. (2002). Nutritive Value of Foods, U.S Department of Agriculture.
4. Nutritional information from the Nutritional label of the packaged food product.

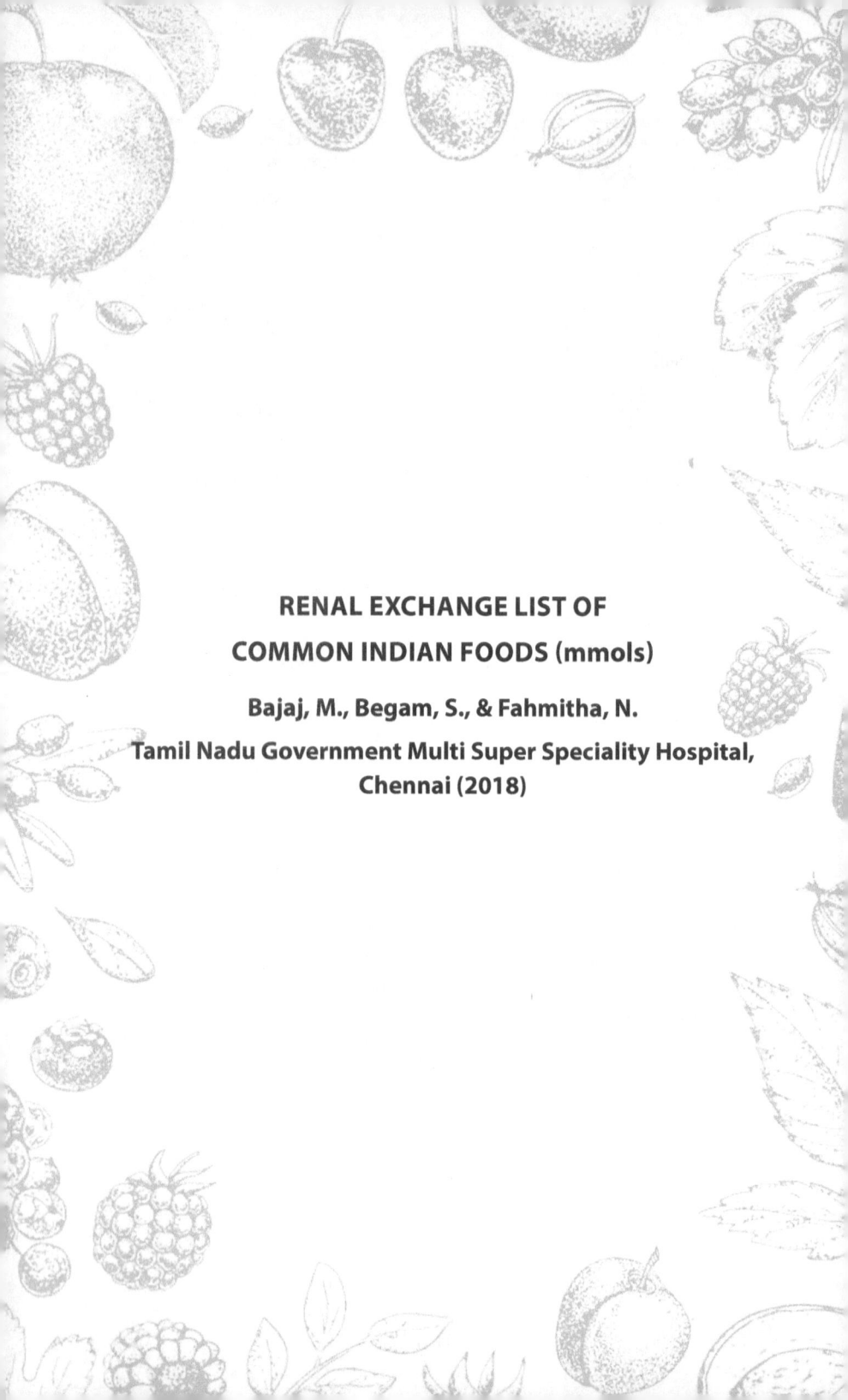

RENAL EXCHANGE LIST OF
COMMON INDIAN FOODS (mmols)

Bajaj, M., Begam, S., & Fahmitha, N.

Tamil Nadu Government Multi Super Speciality Hospital, Chennai (2018)

Food Ingredient	Raw Weight (g)	Sodium (mmol)	Potassium (mmol)	Phosphorus (mmol)
Cereal				
Barley	100	0	7	59
Dosa flour (dry)	100	34	9	60
Idly flour (dry)	100	34	9	60
Quinoa	100	0	12	71
Rice flakes (dry)	100	0	4	65
Rice, Parboiled milled	100	0	4	47
Rice, raw milled	100	0	3	32
Wheat flour, refined	100	0	4	37
Wheat, Semolina (dry)	100	0	7	40
Wheat, Vermicelli (dry)	100	0	4	33
Whole wheat flour	100	0	8	105
Millet				
Bajra	100	0	9	96
Jowar	100	0	8	91
Ragi	100	0	11	70
Samai	100	0	3	43
Varagu	100	0	2	34
Pulse				
Bengal gram, dhal	100	1	25	108
Bengal gram, whole	100	1	24	89
Black gram, dhal	100	1	30	125
Black gram, whole	100	1	28	115
Cow pea,white	100	1	32	126
Green gram, dhal	100	0	33	139
Green gram, whole	100	1	30	118
Horse gram, whole	100	1	27	99
Peas dry	100	1	24	111
Rajma,red	100	0	34	136
Red gram, dhal	100	1	36	109
Soyabean, white	100	0	42	165

(Contd.)

Food Ingredient	Raw Weight (g)	Sodium (mmol)	Potassium (mmol)	Phosphorus (mmol)
Vegetable Group A (Green Leafy Vegetables)				
Agathi leaves	100	1	17	18
Amaranth leaves,green	100	1	15	24
Cabbage, Green	100	1	6	10
Cauliflower leaves	100	1	10	21
Drumstick leaves	100	0	10	36
Fenugreek leaves	100	2	6	18
Lettuce	100	1	7	15
Mustard leaves	100	1	10	24
Ponnaganni	100	2	12	19
Radish leaves	100	1	8	17
Spinach	100	2	16	11
Group B (Roots & Tubers)				
Beetroot	100	3	8	12
Carrot, Orange	100	2	7	14
Colacasia	100	0	13	27
Potato, brown skin big	100	0	14	14
Sweet potato, Pink skin	100	1	8	13
Tapioca	100	0	7	14
Yam,elephant	100	1	13	14
Group C (Other Vegetables)				
Ash gourd	100	0	10	10
Beans scarlet tender	100	0	4	21
Bittergourd, jagged, teethridges, elongate	100	1	8	15
Bottle gourd, elongate, pale green	100	0	3	5
Brinjal all varieties	100	0	6	11
Cauliflower	100	1	8	16
Cucumber, green elongate	100	0	5	9

Food Ingredient	Raw Weight (g)	Sodium (mmol)	Potassium (mmol)	Phosphorus (mmol)
Ladies finger	100	0	7	19
Plantain flower	100	0	13	16
Ridge gourd	100	0	3	11
Snake gourd, long, pale green	100	0	3	8
Tomato, Green	100	1	6	8
Tomato, red ripe local	100	0	5	6
Zucchini,green	100	0	5	7
Fruit				
Apple, big	100	0	3	3
Banana, ripe, poovam	100	0	9	11
Custard apple	100	0	7	14
Dates, processed	100	0	7	11
Gooseberry	100	0	6	7
Grapes, green round seeded	100	0	4	7
Guava, white flesh	100	0	7	8
Jackfruit, ripe	100	0	7	8
Jambufruit, ripe	100	0	3	3
Mango, ripe, banganapalli	100	0	4	4
Musk melon, orange flesh	100	1	5	6
Orange, pulp	100	0	4	4
Papaya, ripe	100	0	4	6
Pear	100	0	3	2
Pineapple	100	0	4	5
Plum	100	0	4	5
Sapota	100	0	7	7
Strawberry	100	0	4	9
Sweet lime, pulp	100	0	5	7
Tamarind, pulp	100	1	21	38
Watermelon, dark green	100	0	3	4

(Contd.)

Food Ingredient	Raw Weight (g)	Sodium (mmol)	Potassium (mmol)	Phosphorus (mmol)
Milk & Milk Products				
Buttermilk (cow's milk)*	100 ml	0	NA	10
Curd*	100 g	1	3	31
Milk, whole, Buffalo	100 ml	1	3	29
Milk, whole, Cow	100 ml	1	3	32
Paneer	100 g	1	2	110
Skimmed milk powder*	100 g	0	NA	333
Skimmed milk*	100 ml	0	NA	30
Egg & Animal Meat				
Beef, chops	100	1	10	70
Chicken,poultry, breast, skinless	100	2	8	59
Egg, poultry, whole, raw	100	5	4	62
Goat, chops	100	2	9	65
Marine Fish				
Anchovy (Nethili)	100	9	7	82
Paarai (Jack fish)	100	2	10	95
Pomfret, black	100	3	8	65
Prawns , big	100	37	7	79
Salmon fish	100	1	9	70
Vanjaram (Seer fish)	100	2	12	101
Condiments & Spices				
Asafoetida	100	1	6	23
Cardamom, green	100	1	32	44
Chillies, green all varieties	100	0	9	17
Chillies, red	100	1	58	93
Cloves	100	8	37	28
Coriander leaves	100	2	14	22
Coriander seed	100	1	38	98

Food Ingredient	Raw Weight (g)	Sodium (mmol)	Potassium (mmol)	Phosphorus (mmol)
Cumin seed	100	5	48	127
Curry leaves	100	1	15	28
Fenugreek seed	100	2	23	145
Garlic, big clove	100	0	11	40
Ginger,fresh	100	0	10	15
Mint leaves	100	1	14	22
Omum	100	1	43	110
Onion, big	100	0	4	11
Onion, small	100	0	4	13
Pepper, black	100	1	38	48
Poppy seeds	100	1	17	268
Turmeric powder	100	1	61	92
Nuts & Oil Seeds				
Almond	100	0	18	149
Cashew	100	0	16	167
Coconut, kernel, fresh	100	0	6	23
Groundnut	100	1	17	130
Mustard seed	100	0	18	238
Pistachio nut	100	0	27	179
Walnut	100	0	12	133
Sugars				
Honey*	100	NA	NA	6
Jaggery	100	1	13	25
Sago*	100	NA	NA	NA
Sugar**	100	N	N	NA

Note:

- Source :Retrieved From: IFCT (2017), NIN* (1989) & USDA** (2002)
- Zero- "0" Below detectable limit
- Abbreviations: NA-Not Available, N – Negligible

Processed Foods	Raw Weight (g)	Sodium (mmol)	Potassium (mmol)	Phosphorus (mmol)
PROCESSED CEREALS				
Modern sweet bread	100	NA	NA	NA
Quaker oats	100	N	NA	NA
Cornflakes, Kellogg's	100	N	NA	NA
Tetrapack Juice				
Tropicana - Orange	100	1	2	NA
Real – Pomegranate	100	2	1	NA
Carbonated Beverages				
Pepsi	100	N	NA	NA
Mount dew	100	1	NA	NA
Pickles				
777 Mango pickle	100	202	NA	NA
Instant Soup				
Knorr mixed vegetable soup	100	161	NA	NA
Chings sweet corn veg soup	100	249	NA	NA
Chocolate				
Diary milk	100	7	NA	NA
Noodles				
Maggi noodles	100	56	NA	NA
Knorr mast masala noodles	100	83	NA	NA
Appalam				
Binduappalam	100	N	NA	NA
Popcorn				
Act II popcorn (Golden sizzle)	100	N	NA	NA
American garden - Cheese popcorn	100	42	NA	NA

Processed Foods	Raw Weight (g)	Sodium (mmol)	Potassium (mmol)	Phosphorus (mmol)
Biscuit				
Cadbury original Oreo sandwich biscuit	100	22	NA	NA
Ketchup				
Kissan ketchup	100	39	NA	NA
Jam				
Kissan jam	100	1	NA	NA
Sauce				
Jerrys chilli sauce	100	204	5	NA
Milk Products				
Britannia cheese cubes	100	63	NA	195
Nestle milkmaid	100	6	NA	NA
Amul butter	100	36	NA	NA
Malt Beverage				
Horlicks	100	17	12	93
Ovaltin	100	4	NA	NA
Squash and Instant Drink Mix				
Kissan orange squash	100	3	1	NA
Tang orange instant drink mix	100	1	NA	NA
Namkeen				
Kurkure aloo bhujia	100	40	NA	NA
Haldiram's bhujia sev	100	34	NA	NA

RENAL SUPPLEMENTS (Oral Nutrition/Enteral)	Raw Weight (g)	Sodium (mmol)	Potassium (mmol)	Phosphorus (mmol)
Essential Renal	100	1	3	58
Fresubin HP	100	6	6	47
Fresubin LP	100	5	3	64
Kabipro	100	10	18	130
Nepro HP	100	6	7	64
Nepro LP	100	7	8	65
Proseventy	100	34	7	233
Real HP	100	12	12	67
Pentasure Renal	100	5	4	64
Pentasure DLS	100	6	6	48
Resource Renal	100	11	11	48
Resource Dialysis	100	12	12	57

Note:

- RETRIEVED FROM: Nutritional information from the Nutritional label of the packaged food product
- Nutrient values have been rounded off to the nearest number
- Since the sodium, potassium, phosphorus content for fats & oils are below detectable amounts, the sodium, potassium, phosphorus content for these is considered as negligible.
- Abbreviations: NA – Not available, N – Negligible

SODIUM CONTENT OF FOODS

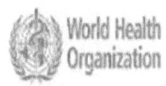

World Health Organization

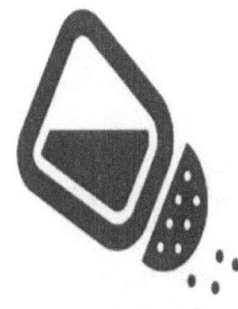

Reducing salt intake to
less than 5 grams per day
(about 1 teaspoon)

can start with comparing labels
at supermarkets and **choosing products
with less sodium**

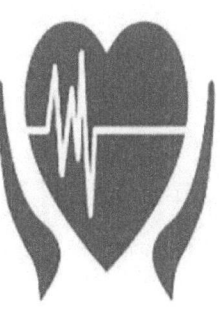

#LessSalt

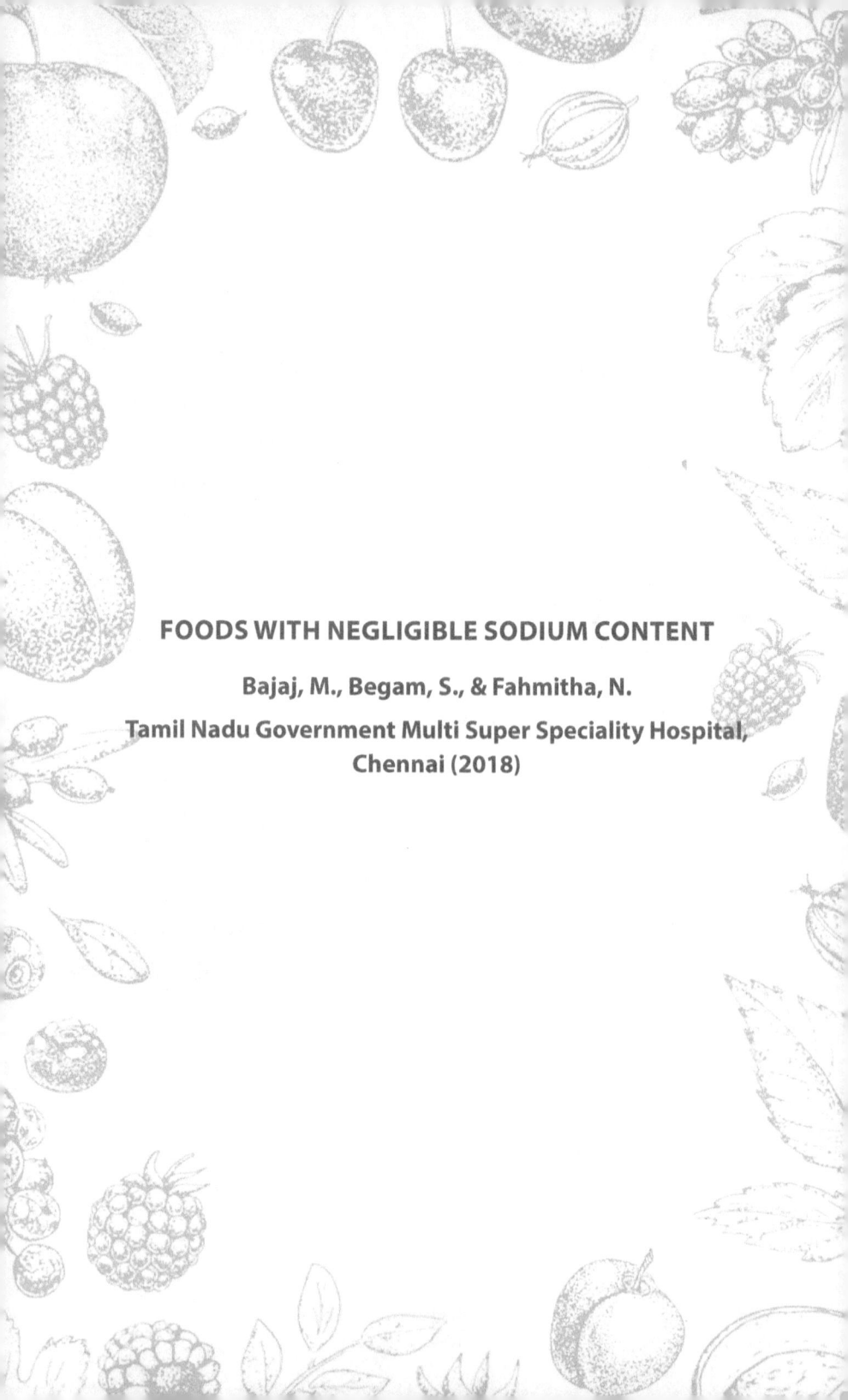

FOODS WITH NEGLIGIBLE SODIUM CONTENT

Bajaj, M., Begam, S., & Fahmitha, N.

Tamil Nadu Government Multi Super Speciality Hospital, Chennai (2018)

SODIUM AND SALT MEASUREMENT EQUIVALENT

- Sodium chloride is approximately 40% (39.3%) Sodium and 60% chloride.
- To convert a specific weight of Sodium chloride to its Sodium equivalent, multiply the weight by 0.393.
- Sodium also is measured in milliequivalents (mEq).
- To convert milligrams of Sodium to mEq, divide by by the atomic weight of 23.
- To convert Sodium to Sodium chloride (salt), multiply by 2.54.
- Millimoles (mmol) and Milliequivalents (mEq) of sodium are the same.

For example:

1tsp of salt = approximately 6g NaCl.

6096 mg NaCl * 0.393 = 2396 mg Na (approx.2400mg)

2396 mg Na/23 = 104 mEq Na

1g Na = 1000 mg/23 = 43 mEq or mmol

1tsp of salt = 2400 mg or 104 mEq Na

Reference

1. Mahan, L.K., &Raymond, J.L. (Eds.).(2016). *Krause's food & the nutrition care process,* (14[th]ed.). St.Louis, Missouri:Elsevier.

FOOD LABELLING GUIDE FOR SODIUM

Sodium – free	Less than 5mg per standard serving; cannot contain any sodium chloride
Very low sodium	35 mg or less per standard serving
Low sodium	140mg or less per standard serving
Reduced sodium	At least 25% less sodium per standard serving than in the regular food
Light in sodium	50% less sodium per standard serving than in the regular food
Unsalted, without added salt, or no salt added	No salt added during processing; the product it resembles is normally processed with salt
Lightly salted	50% less added sodium than is normally added; product must state "not a low-sodium food" if that criterion is not met.

Reference

1. Mahan, L.K., &Raymond, J.L. (Eds.). (2016). *Krause's food & the nutrition care process*, (14thed.). St.Louis, Missouri: Elsevier.

NEGLIGIBLE SODIUM CONTENT
<5mg / <0.21mmol
Sodium per 100g (Edible Portion)

Cereals	Roots and Tubers	Fruits	Condiments and Spices
Chapathi, whole wheat flour	Colocasia	Apple, Big	Chillies, green all varieties
Quinoa	Potato, brown skin, big	Banana, ripe, Poovam	Onion, small
Rice flakes(dry)		Custard Apple	
Rice, Parboiled milled	**Other Vegetables**	Dates, Processed	**Sugars**
Rice, raw milled	Ash gourd	Gooseberry	Sugar
Wheat, flour refined	Beans scarlet, tender	Grapes, green round seeded	
Wheat, Semolina (dry)	Bottle gourd, elongate, pale green	Guava, white flesh	**Processed Products**
Wheat, Vermicelli (dry)	Brinjal all varieties	Jackfruit, ripe	Act II popcorn (Golden sizzle)
	Ridge gourd	Jambu fruit, ripe	Bindu appalam
Millets	Zucchini, green	Mango, ripe, banganapalli	Kellogg's cornflakes
Bajra		Orange, pulp	Quaker oats
Jowar	**Nuts**	Pear	
Ragi	Almond	Pineapple	
Samai	Mustard seed	Plum	
Varagu	Walnut	Sapota	
PULSES		Strawberry	
Soyabean, White		Sweet lime, Pulp	
		Watermelon, dark green	

Source: IFCT (2017), NIN (1989) & Nutritional information from the Nutritional label of the packaged food product

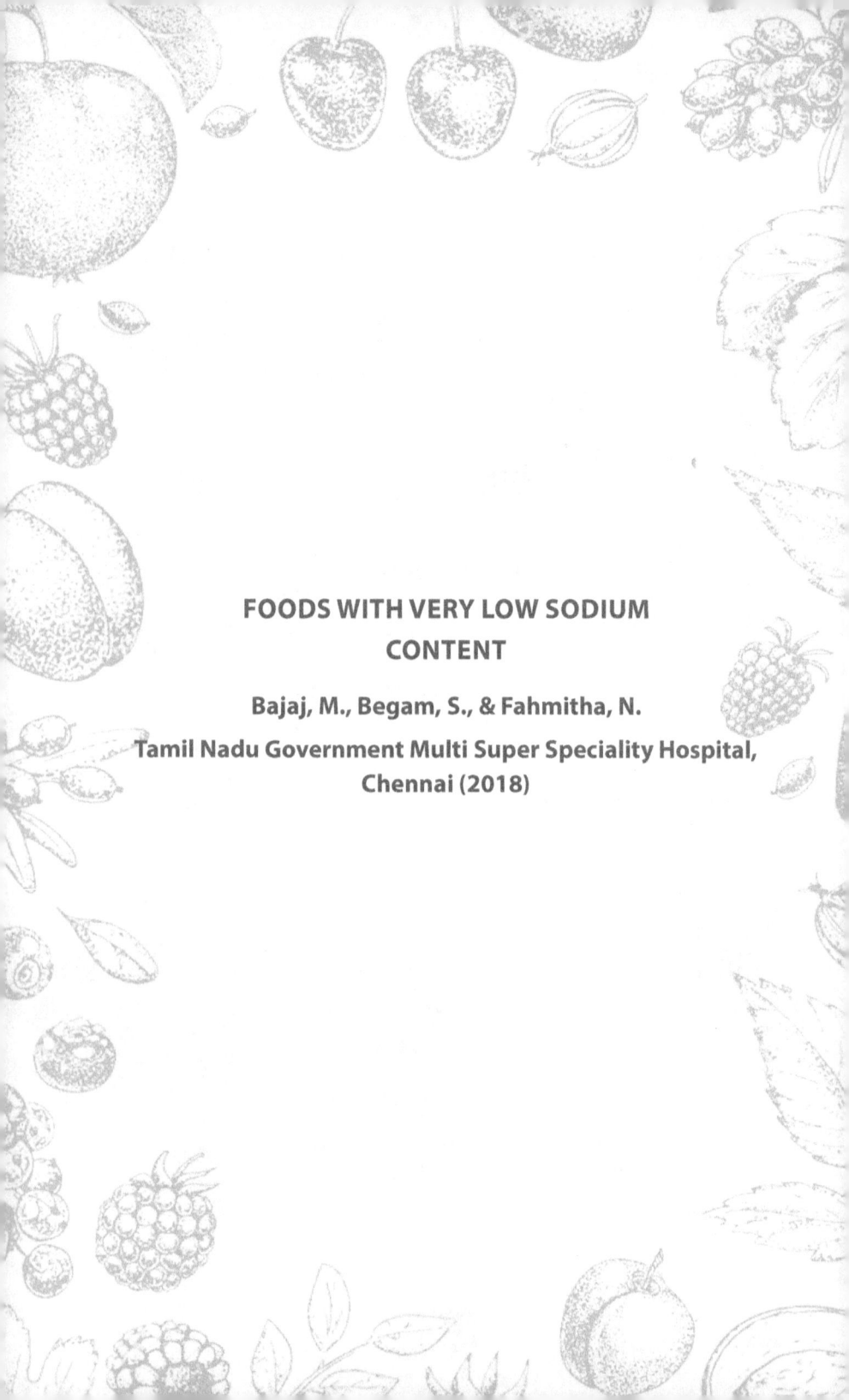

FOODS WITH VERY LOW SODIUM CONTENT

Bajaj, M., Begam, S., & Fahmitha, N.

Tamil Nadu Government Multi Super Speciality Hospital, Chennai (2018)

VERY LOW SODIUM CONTENT
5-35mg / 0.21-1.5mmol
Sodium per 100g (Edible Portion)

Cereals	Fruits	Other Vegetables	Condiments and Spices	Nuts
Barley	Musk melon , orange flesh	Bitter gourd, jagged, teeth ridges, elongate	Asafoetida	Cashew
Millets	Papaya, ripe	Cauliflower	Cardamom, green	Coconut, kernel, fresh
Jowar	Tamarind, pulp	Cucumber, green elongate	Chillies, red	Groundnut
Pulses	**Green Leafy Vegetables**	Ladies finger	Coriander seed	Pistachio nut
Bengal gram, Dhal	Agathi leaves	Plantain flower	Curry leaves	**Sugars**
Bengal gram, Whole	Amaranth leaves, green	Snake gourd, long, pale green	Garlic, big clove	Jaggery
Black gram, Dhal	Cabbage, Green	Tomato, Green	Ginger, fresh	**Processed Products**
Black gram, whole	Cauliflower leaves	Tomato, red ripe local	Mint leaves	Kissan Jam
Cow pea, white	Drumstick leaves	**Milk**	Omum	Mount dew
Green gram, Dhal	Lettuce	Curd*	Onion, big	Pepsi
Green gram, Whole	Mustard leaves	Milk, whole, Cow	Pepper, black	Tang orange instant drink mix
Horse gram, Whole	**Roots and Tubers**	Milk, whole, Buffalo	Poppy seeds	
Peas dry	Sweet potato, Pink skin	Paneer	Turmeric powder	Tropicana - Orange
Rajmah , red	Tapioca	**Meat**	**Marine**	
Red gram, Dhal	Yam, elephant	Beef, chops	Salmon fish	
			Vanjaram (Seer Fish)	

Source: IFCT (2017), NIN (1989)&Nutritional information from the Nutritional label of the packaged food product

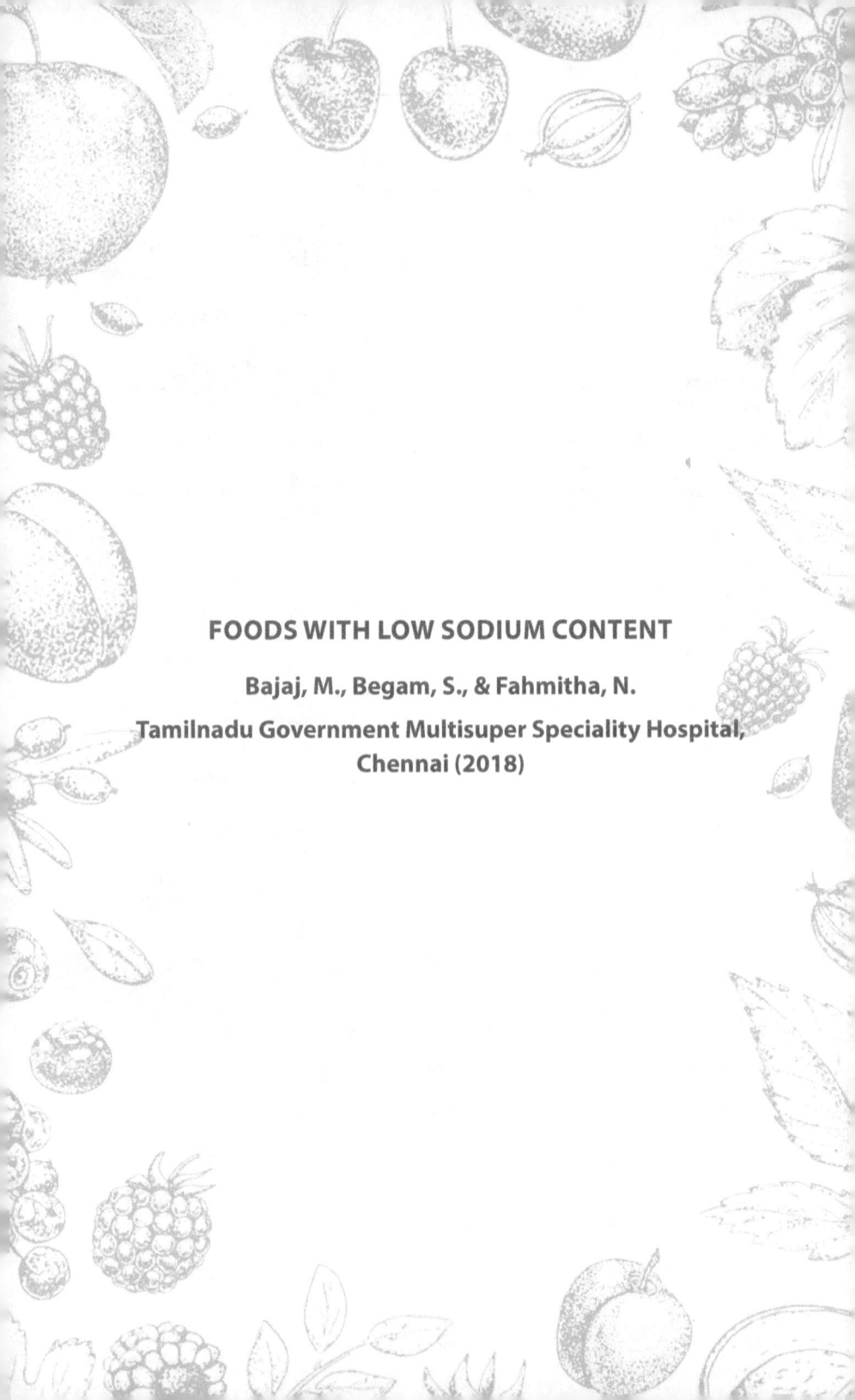

FOODS WITH LOW SODIUM CONTENT

Bajaj, M., Begam, S., & Fahmitha, N.

Tamilnadu Government Multisuper Speciality Hospital, Chennai (2018)

LOW SODIUM CONTENT
35-140 mg /1.5-6.08 mmol
Sodium per 100 g (Edible Portion)

Green Leafy Vegetables	Meat	Processed Products
Fenugreek leaves	Chicken, poultry, breast, skinless	Kissan orange squash
Ponnaganni	Egg, poultry, whole raw	Ovaltin
Radish leaves	Goat, chops	Real - Pomegranate
Spinach	**Marine**	
Roots and Tubers	Paarai	
Carrot, Orange	Pomfret, black	
Beetroot	**Condiments and Spices**	
	Coriander leaves	
	Cumin seed	
	Fenugreek seed	

Source: IFCT (2017), NIN (1989)&Nutritional information from the Nutritional label of the packaged food product.

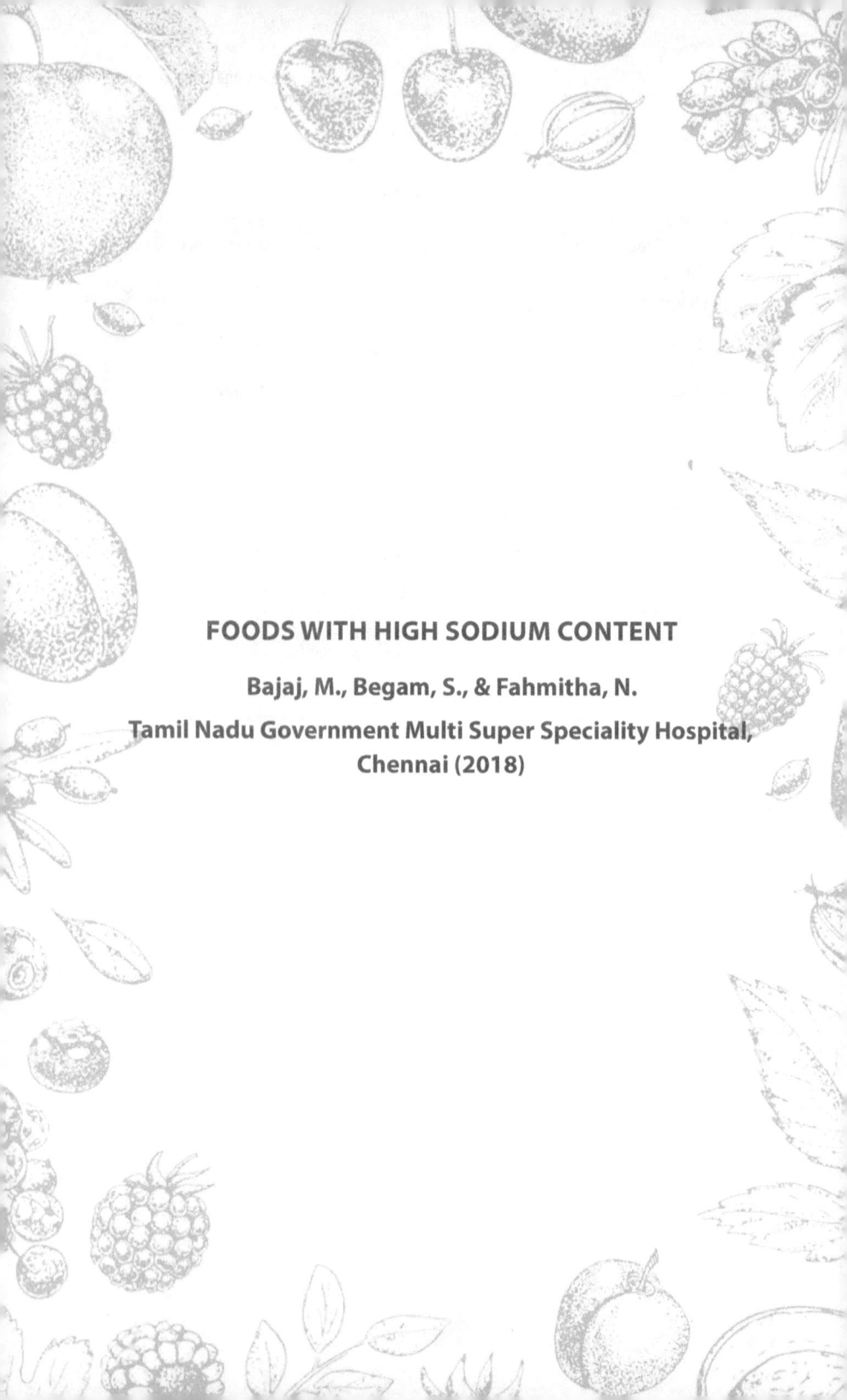

FOODS WITH HIGH SODIUM CONTENT

Bajaj, M., Begam, S., & Fahmitha, N.

Tamil Nadu Government Multi Super Speciality Hospital, Chennai (2018)

HIGH SODIUM CONTENT
>140mg / >6.08mmol
Sodium per 100g (Edible Portion)

Cereal	Processed Products
Dosa flour (dry)	777 Mango pickle
Idly flour(dry)	American garden - Cheese popcorn
	Amul butter
Marine	Britannia cheese cubes
Anchovy (Nethili)	Cadbury original Oreo sandwich biscuit
Prawns , big	Chings sweet corn veg soup
	Diary milk
Condiments and Spices	Haldiram's bhujia sev
Cloves	Horlicks
	Jerry's chilli sauce
	Kissan ketchup
	Knorr mast masala noodles
	Knorr mixed vegetable soup
	Kurkure aloo bhujia
	Maggi noodles
	Nestle milkmaid

Source: IFCT (2017), NIN (1989) &Nutritional information from the Nutritional label of the packaged food product

POTASSIUM CONTENT OF FOODS

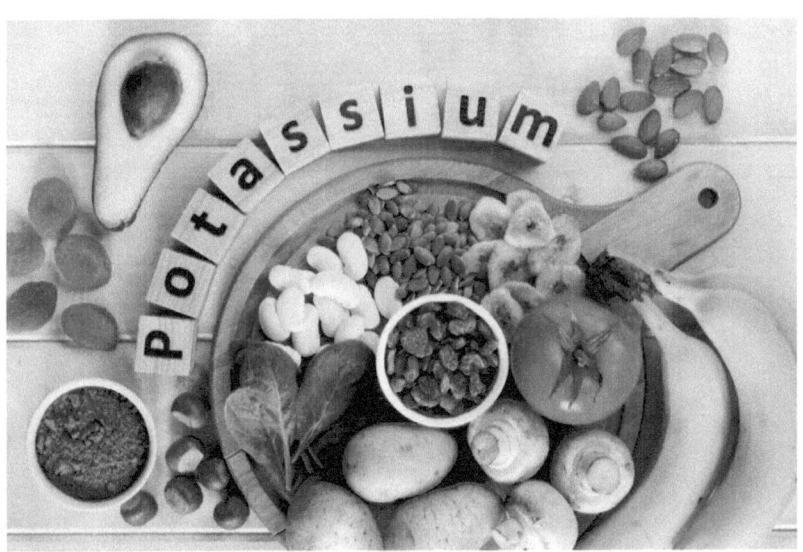

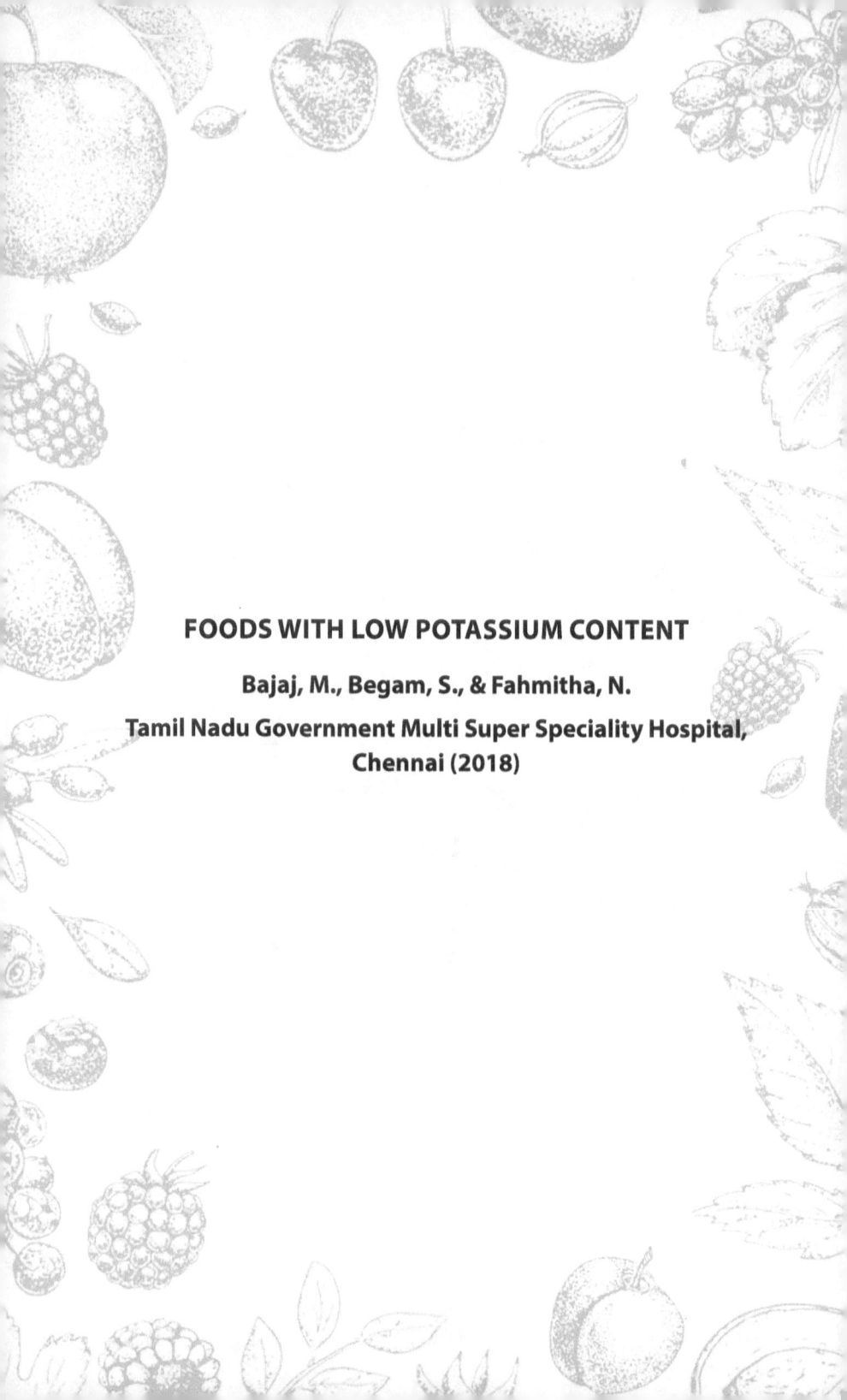

FOODS WITH LOW POTASSIUM CONTENT

Bajaj, M., Begam, S., & Fahmitha, N.

Tamil Nadu Government Multi Super Speciality Hospital, Chennai (2018)

LOW POTASSIUM CONTENT
<100mg / <2.56 mmol
Potassium per 100g (Edible Portion)

Millet	Sugars
Jowar	Sugar
Pearl millet (Bajra)	**Processed Products**
Samai	Kissan orange squash
Varagu	Real – Pomegranate
Milk	Tropicana - Orange
Paneer	

Source: IFCT (2017), NIN (1989) &Nutritional information from the Nutritional label of the packaged food product

Kindly note the details that processed foods even if found low in Potassium, do not warrant inclusion in patients.

The details are provide for information only.

FOODS WITH MEDIUM POTASSIUM CONTENT

Bajaj, M., Begam, S., & Fahmitha, N.

Tamil Nadu Government Multi Super Speciality Hospital, Chennai (2018)

MEDIUM POTASSIUM CONTENT
100-200mg / 2.56-5.12mmol
Potassium per 100g (Edible Portion)

Cereals	Fruits	Milk
Rice flakes (dry)	Apple, Big	Curd*
Rice, Parboiled milled	Grapes, green round seeded	Milk, whole, buffalo
Rice, raw milled	Jambu fruit, ripe	Milk, whole, cow
Wheat flour, refined	Mango, ripe, Banganapalli	
Wheat, Vermicelli (dry)	Orange, pulp	**Meat**
Millets	Papaya, ripe	Egg, poultry, whole raw
Finger millet (Ragi)	Pear	
Other Vegetables	Pineapple	**Condiments and Spices**
Beans scarlet tender	Plum	Onion, small
Bottle gourd, elongate, pale green	Strawberry	Onion, big
Cucumber, green elongate	Sweet lime, Pulp	
Ridge gourd	Watermelon, dark green	**Processed Products**
Snake gourd, long, pale green		Jerry's chilli sauce
Zucchini, green		

Source: IFCT (2017), NIN (1989)&Nutritional information from the Nutritional label of the packaged food product

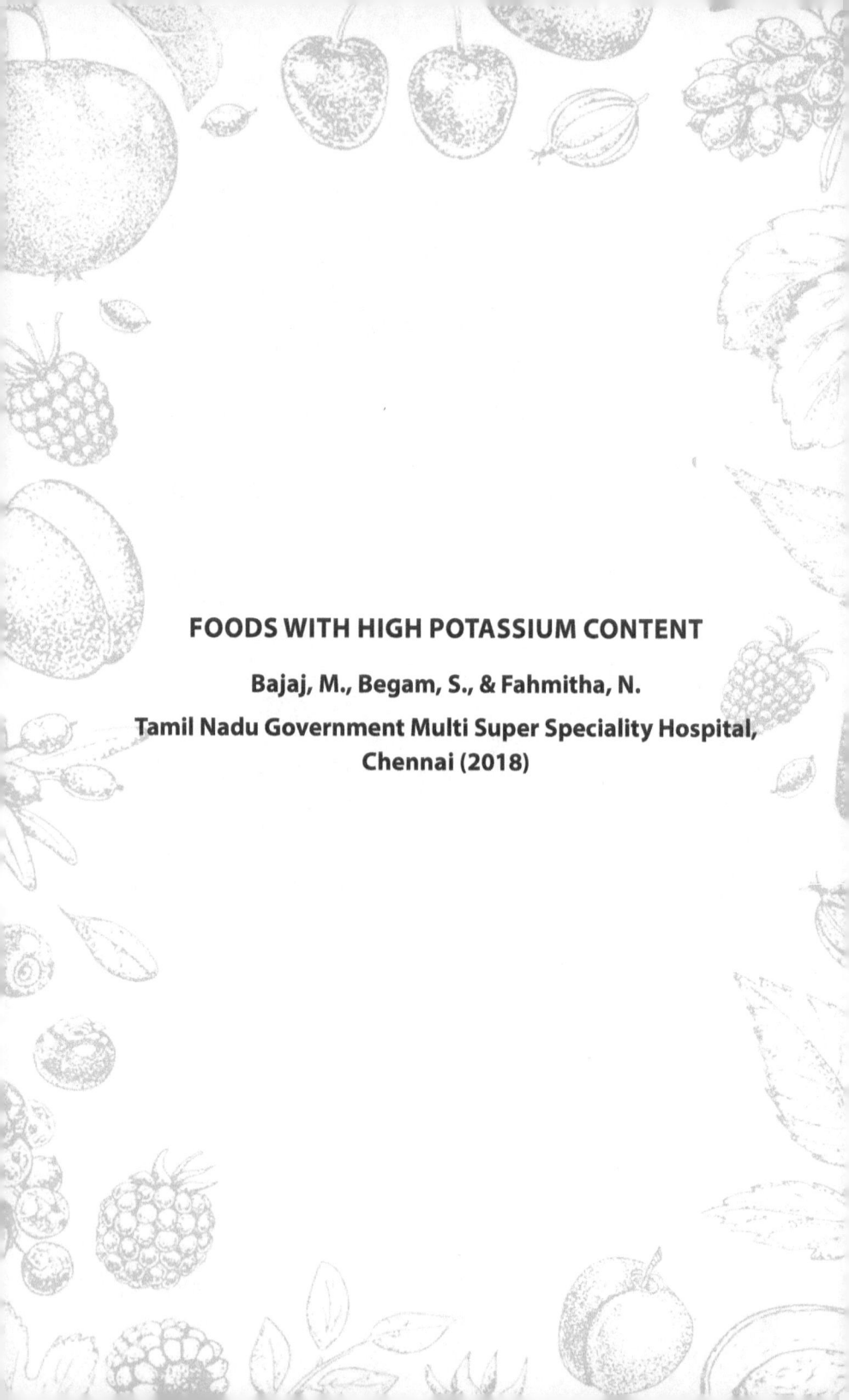

FOODS WITH HIGH POTASSIUM CONTENT

Bajaj, M., Begam, S., & Fahmitha, N.

Tamil Nadu Government Multi Super Speciality Hospital, Chennai (2018)

HIGH POTASSIUM CONTENT
>200 mg / >5.12 mmol
Potassium per 100 g (Edible Portion)

Cereals	Green Leafy Vegetables	Other Vegetables	Marine	Condiments and Spices
Barley	Agathi leaves	Ash gourd	Anchovy (Nethili)	Asafoetida
Dosa flour (dry)	Amaranth leaves, green	Bitter gourd, jagged, teeth ridges, elongate	Paarai	Cardamom, green
Idly flour (dry)	Cabbage, Green		Pomfret, black	Chillies, green all varieties
Quinoa	Cauliflower leaves	Brinjal all varieties	Prawns , big	Chillies, red
Wheat, Semolina (dry)	Drumstick leaves	Cauliflower	Salmon fish	Cloves
Whole wheat flour	Fenugreek leaves	Ladies finger	Vanjaram (Seer)	Coriander leaves
Pulses	Lettuce	Plantain flower	**Nuts**	Coriander seed
Bengal gram, Dhal	Mustard leaves	Tomato, Green	Almond	Cumin seed
Bengal gram, Whole	Ponnaganni	Tomato, red ripe local	Cashew	Curry leaves
Black gram, Dhal	Radish leaves	Ash gourd	Coconut, kernel, fresh	Fenugreek seed
Black gram, whole	Spinach	**Fruits**	Groundnut	Garlic, big clove
Cow pea, white	**Roots and Tubers**	Banana, ripe, Poovam	Mustard seed	Ginger, fresh
Green gram, Dhal	Beetroot	Custard Apple	Pistachio nut	Mint leaves
Green gram, Whole	Carrot, Orange	Dates, Processed	Walnut	Omum
Horse gram, Whole	Colocasia	Gooseberry	**Processed Products**	Pepper, black
Peas dry	Potato, brown skin big	Guava, white flesh	Horlicks	Poppy seeds

(Contd.)

HIGH POTASSIUM CONTENT
>200 mg / >5.12 mmol
Potassium per 100 g (Edible Portion)

Pulses and Whole grams	Roots and Tubers	Fruits	Condiments and Spices
Rajmah, red	Sweet potato, Pink skin	Jackfruit, ripe	Turmeric powder
Red gram, Dhal	Tapioca	Musk melon, orange flesh	
Soyabean, White	Yam, elephant	Sapota	
Meat	**Sugars**	Tamarind, pulp	
Beef chops	Jaggery		
Chicken, poultry, breast, skinless			
Goat chops			

Source: IFCT (2017), NIN (1989) & Nutritional information from the Nutritional label of the packaged food product

FRUIT EXCHANGE WITH LOW POTASSIUM CONTENT

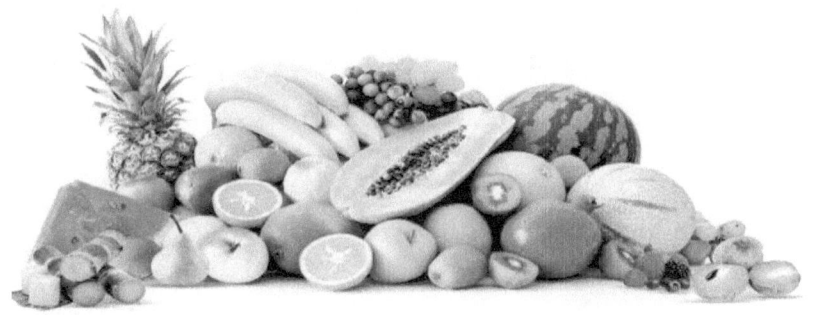

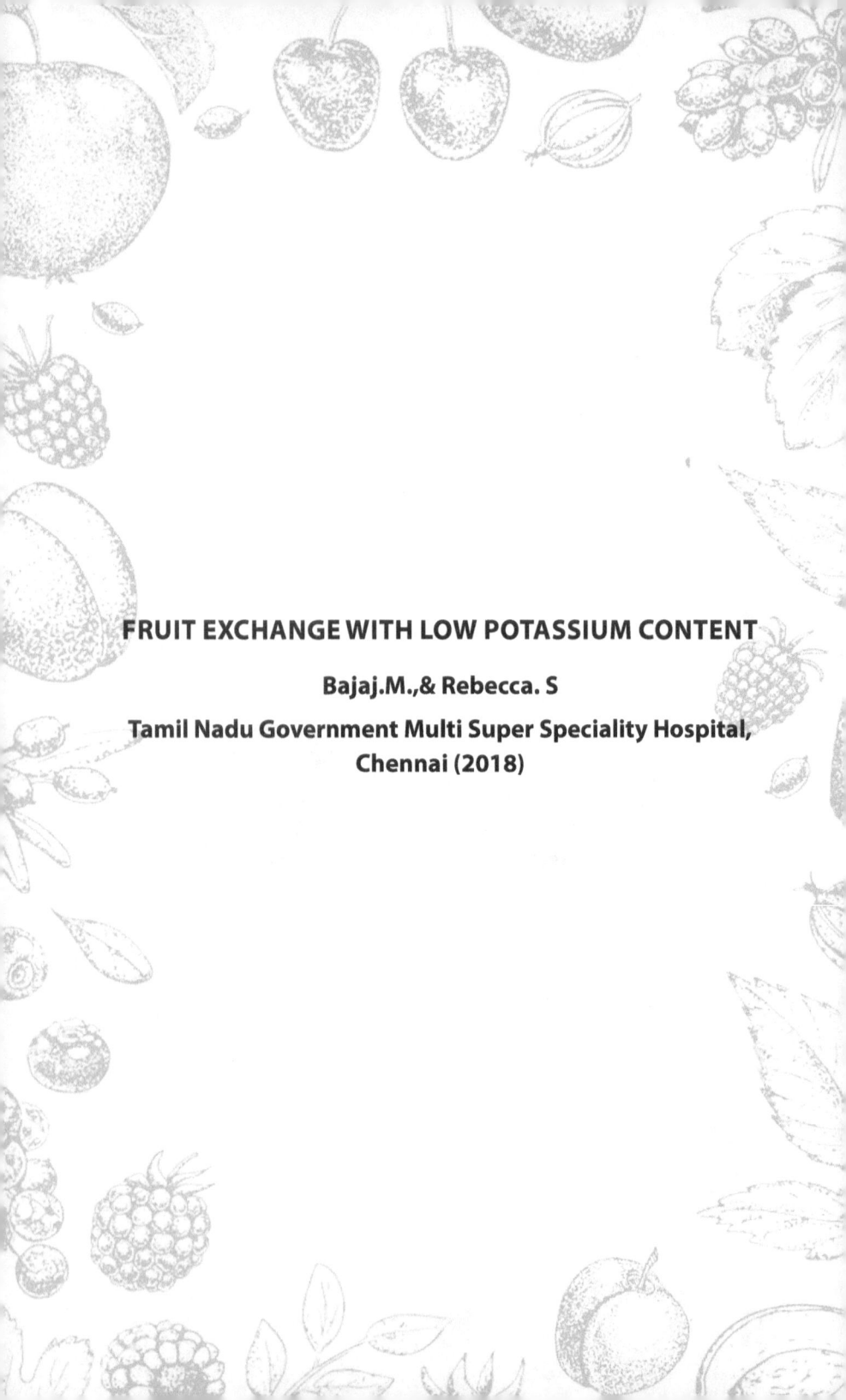

FRUIT EXCHANGE WITH LOW POTASSIUM CONTENT

Bajaj.M.,& Rebecca. S

Tamil Nadu Government Multi Super Speciality Hospital, Chennai (2018)

LOW POTASSIUM FRUIT EXCHANGE
<100mg /serving size

Fruit	Quantity Edible Portion (g)	Portion Size
Amla(Goose berry- Big)	44	6-7nos
Apple, big	85	3/4 apple
Banana, poovam	30	1/4 = 2"
Custard apple	35	1 medium
Dates,processed	12	2 nos
Grapes, seedless, oval, black	41	15- 20 nos
Guava, white flesh	35	1 piece
Jackfruit	35	2 nos
Jambu	96	20 nos
Mango, ripe, banganapalli	70	1/2 medium size
Orange, pulp	60	1/2 medium
Papaya	60	2 thin slice
Pear	95	1 medium
Pineapple	70	3/4 thin slice
Plum	60	2-3 nos
Sapota	35	3 piece
Strawberry	70	1/2 cup (5-6 nos)
Sweet lime	55	1/2 medium
Watermelon, pale green	78	1 slice

References

1. Longvah, T., Ananthan, R., Bhaskarachary, K., &Venkaiah, K. (2017). Indian Food Composition Tables, India, Hyderabad: National Institute of Nutrition.

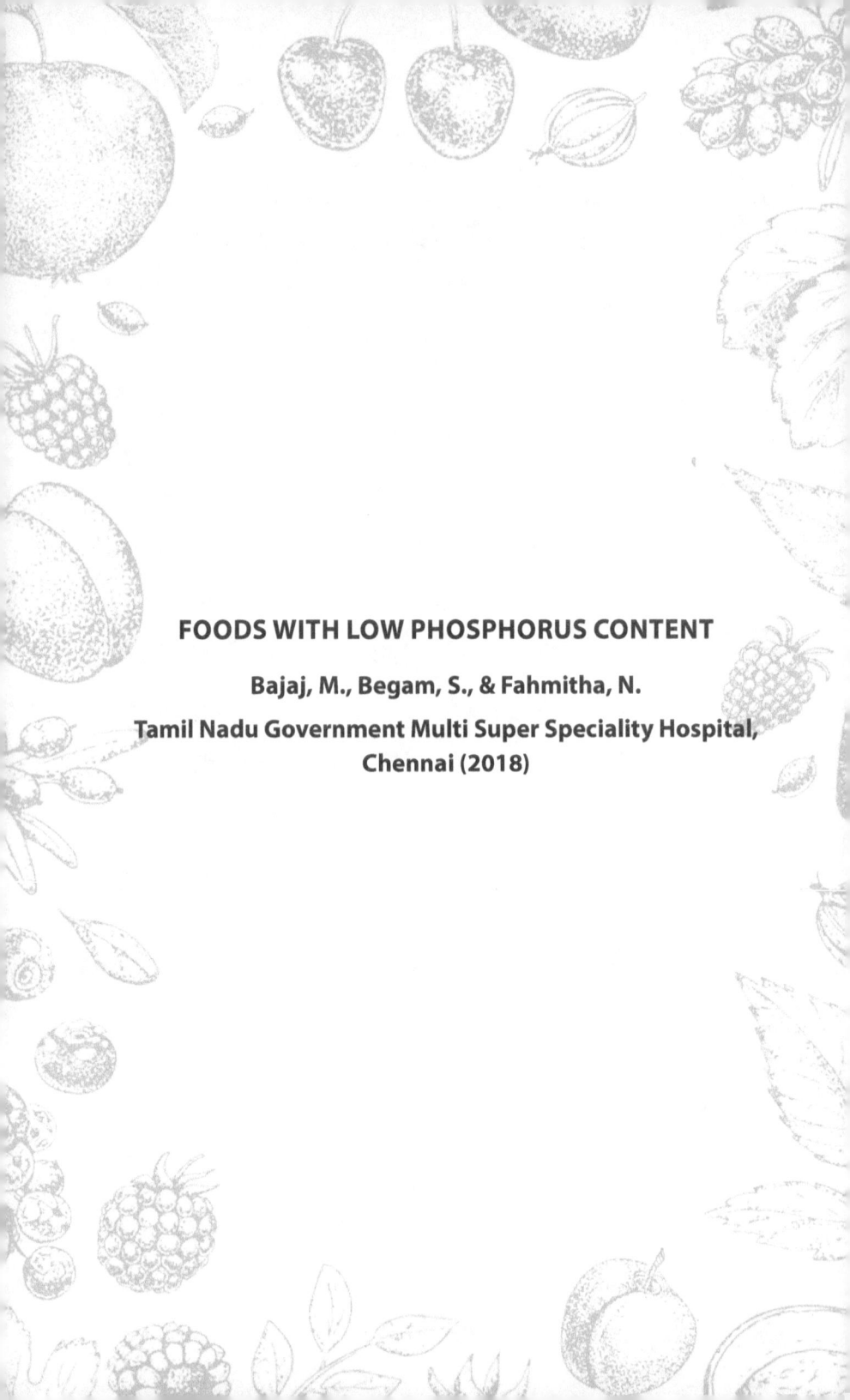

FOODS WITH LOW PHOSPHORUS CONTENT

Bajaj, M., Begam, S., & Fahmitha, N.

Tamil Nadu Government Multi Super Speciality Hospital, Chennai (2018)

LOW PHOSPHORUS CONTENT
0-50mg / >16.66mmol
Phosphorus per 100g (Edible Portion)

Green Leafy Vegetables	Roots and Tubers	Fruit Exchange
Cabbage, Green	Beetroot	Apple, Big
Lettuce	Carrot, Orange	Banana, ripe, Poovam
Spinach	Potato, brown skin big	Custard Apple
	Sweet potato, Pink skin	Dates, Processed
Other Vegetables	Tapioca	Gooseberry
Ash gourd	Yam, elephant	Grapes, green round seeded
Bitter gourd, jagged, teeth ridges, elongate		Guava, white flesh
Bottle gourd, elongate, pale green	**Milk**	Jackfruit, ripe
Brinjal all varieties	Buttermilk (cow's milk)*	Jambu fruit, ripe
Cauliflower		Mango, ripe, banganapalli
Cucumber, green elongate	**Condiments and Spices**	Musk melon , orange flesh
Plantain flower	Ginger, fresh	Orange, pulp
Ridge gourd	Onion, big	Papaya, ripe
Snake gourd, long, pale green	Onion, small	Pear
Tomato, Green		Pineapple
Tomato, red ripe local	**Sugar**	Plum
Zucchini, green	Honey*	Sapota
		Strawberry
		Sweetlime, Pulp
		Watermelon, dark green

Source: IFCT (2017) & NIN (1989)*

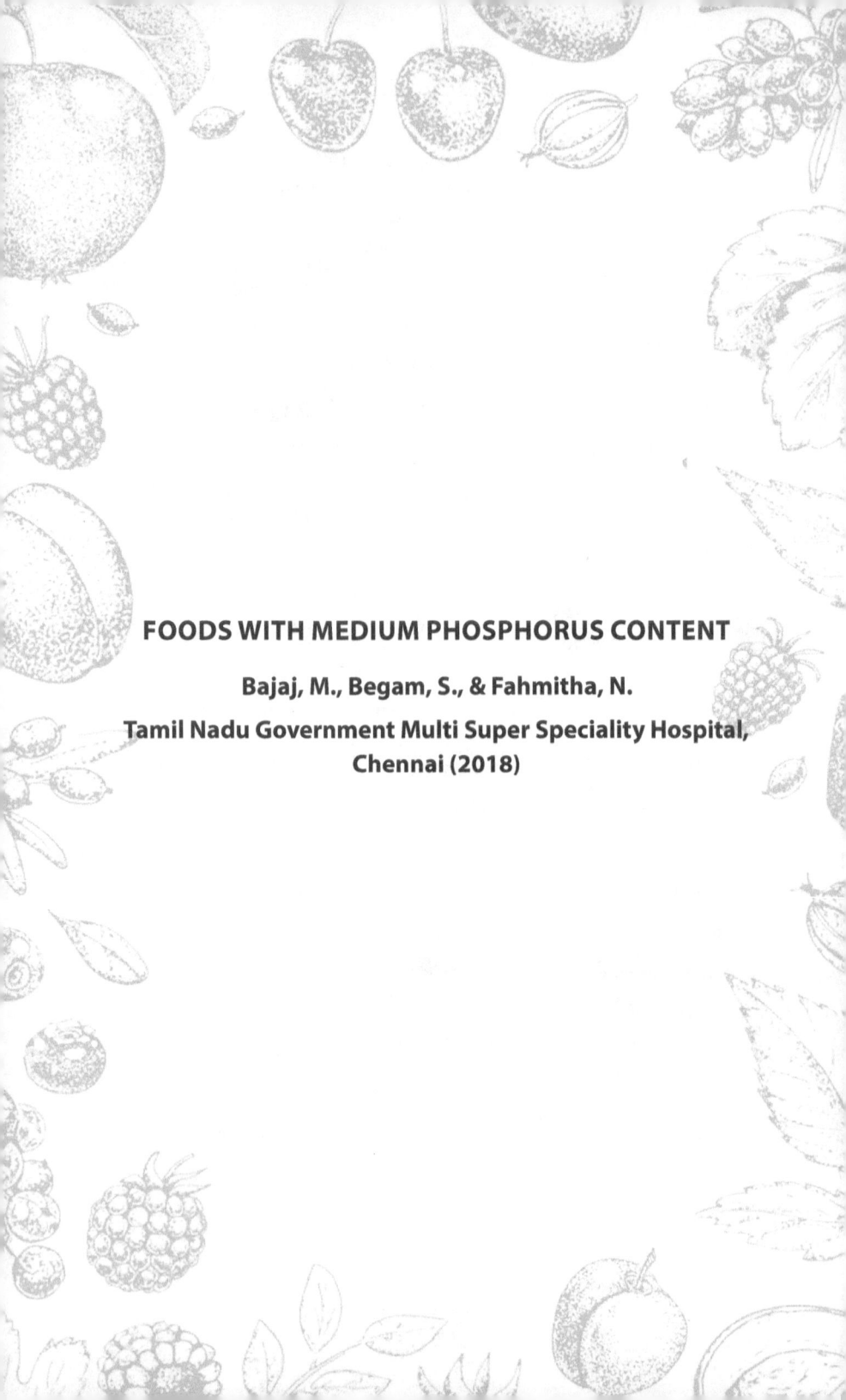

FOODS WITH MEDIUM PHOSPHORUS CONTENT

Bajaj, M., Begam, S., & Fahmitha, N.

Tamil Nadu Government Multi Super Speciality Hospital, Chennai (2018)

MEDIUM PHOSPHORUS CONTENT
50-100 mg / 16.66-33.33 mmol
Phosphorus per 100 g (Edible Portion)

Cereals	Roots and Tubers	Condiments and Spices
Rice, raw milled	Colocasia	Asafoetida
Wheat, Vermicelli (dry)	**Other Vegetables**	Chillies, green, all varieties
Green Leafy Vegetables	Beans scarlet, tender	Cloves
Agathi leaves	Ladies finger	Coriander leaves
Amaranth leaves, green	**Milk**	Curry leaves
Cauliflower leaves	Curd	Mint leaves
Fenugreek leaves	Milk, whole, buffalo	**Nuts**
Mustard leaves	Milk, whole, cow	Coconut, kernel, fresh
Ponnanganni	Skimmed milk	**Sugars**
Radish leaves		Jaggery

Source: IFCT (2017) & NIN (1989)

FOODS WITH HIGH PHOSPHORUS CONTENT

Bajaj, M., Begam, S., & Fahmitha, N.

Tamil Nadu Government Multi Super Speciality Hospital, Chennai (2018)

HIGH PHOSPHORUS CONTENT
>100mg / >33.33 mmol
Phosphorus per 100 g (Edible Portion)

Cereals	Pulses	Marine	Nuts
Barley	Bengal gram, Dhal	Anchovy (Nethili)	Almond
Chapathi, whole wheat flour	Bengal gram, Whole	Paarai (Jack fish)	Cashew nut
Dosa flour (dry)	Black gram, Dhal	Pomfret, black	Groundnut
Idly flour (dry)	Black gram, whole	Prawns , big	Mustard seed
Quinoa	Cow pea, white	Salmon fish	Pistachio nut
Rice flakes	Green gram, Dhal	Vanjaram (Seer fish)	Walnut
Rice, Parboiled milled	Green gram, Whole	**Spices and Condiments**	**Processed Products**
Wheat flour, refined(dry)	Horse gram, Whole	Cardamom, green	Britannia cheese cubes
Wheat, Semolina (dry)	Peas dry	Chillies, red	Horlicks
Millets	Rajma, red	Coriander seed	
Bajra	Red gram, Dhal	Cumin seed	
Jowar	Soyabean, White	Fenugreek seed	
Ragi	**Milk**	Garlic, big clove	
Samai	Paneer	Omum	
Varagu	Skimmed milk powder	Pepper, black	
Green Leafy Vegetables	**Meat**	Poppy seeds	
Drumstick leaves	Beef, chops	Turmeric powder	
Fruits	Chicken breast, skinless		
Tamarind, pulp	Egg, poultry whole raw		
	Goat, chops		

Source: IFCT (2017), NIN (1989) & Nutritional information from the Nutritional label of the packaged food product

References

1. Longvah, T., Ananthan, R., Bhaskarachary, K., &Venkaiah, K. (2017). Indian Food Composition Tables, India, Hyderabad: National Institute of Nutrition.
2. * Gopalan, C., Sastri, B .V. R.,& Balasubramanian, S. C. (1989). Nutritive Value of Indian Foods (Rev.ed.). India, Hyderabad: National Institute of Nutrition.
3. ** Susan, E., Gebhardt., Robin, G., &Thomas. (2002). Nutritive Value of Foods, U.S Department of Agriculture.
4. Nutritional information from the Nutritional label of the packaged food product.

PHOSPHORUS CONTENT IN FOODS

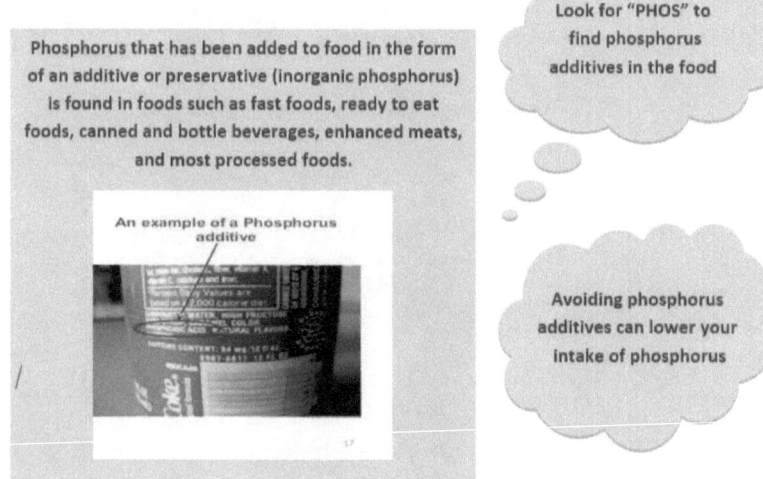

References

1. Phosphorus in CKD (n.d). Retrieved from https://www.kidney.org/atoz/content/phosphorus

TRACK OF NORMAL VALUES

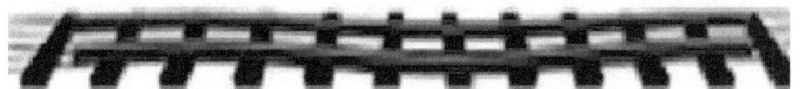

GLUCOSE
(BLOOD SUGAR, FASTING BLOOD SUGAR [FBS])

Reference Range

Fasting blood sugar (FBS): 70-99mg/dL, 3.9-5.5mmol/L

Clinical implication

Increased levels (Hyperglycemia)

Diabetes Mellitus (DM), Cushing syndrome, Acute stress response (Myocardial Infarction(MI), Cerebrovascular accidents [CVA], Burns, Infection, Surgery), Pheochromocytoma, Acromegaly, Gigantism, Chronic renal failure, Glucagonoma, Acute pancreatitis, Pregnancy, Corticosteroid therapy.

Decreased levels (Hypoglycemia)

Pancreatic islet cell carcinoma, Addison disease, Hypothyroidism, Hypopituitarism, Liver disease, Starvation, Insulin overdose.

GLUCOSE, POSTPRANDIAL
(2- HOUR POSTPRANDIAL GLUCOSE [2 – HOUR PPG])

Reference Range

PPG: <140mg/dl

Clinical implications

Increased Levels

Diabetes Mellitus (DM), Gestational Diabetes Mellitus (GDM), Malnutrition, Hyperthyroidism, Acute Stress Response (Myocardial Infarction (MI), Cerebrovascular Accidents (CVA), Burns, Infection, Surgery), Cushing Syndrome, Pheochromocytoma, Chronic Renal Failure, Glucagonoma, Diuretic Therapy, Corticosteroid Therapy, Liver Disease.

Decreased levels

Insulinoma, Hypothyroidism, Hypopituitarism, Insulin Overdose, Addison Disease.

GLUCOSE TOLERANCE
(GT, ORAL GLUCOSE TOLERANCE TEST [OGTT])

Reference range

Fasting: <110mg/dL, <6.1mmol/L
30 minutes: <200mg/dL, 11.1mmol/L
1 hour: <200mg/dL, 11.1mmol/L
2hours: <140mg/dL, <7.8mmol/L
3hours:70-115mg/dL,<6.4mmol/L

Clinical implications

Increased levels

Diabetes Mellitus, Acute Stress Response (Myocardial Infarction (MI), Cerebrovascular Accidents (CVA), Burns, Infection, Surgery), Cushing Syndrome, Pheochromocytoma, Chronic Renal Failure, Glucagonoma, Diuretic Therapy, Corticosteroid Therapy, Liver Disease, Acute Pancreatitis, Myxedema, Somogyi Response to Hypoglycemia.

GLYCOSYLATED HEMOGLOBIN
(GHB, GLYCO HEMOGLOBIN [GHB], HEMOGLOBIN A1c
[Hba1c] OR [A1c]

Reference range

Adult :< 5.7% (ADA, 2018)

Clinical implications

Increased levels

Newly Diagnosed Diabetes Mellitus, Pregnancy, Non - diabetic Hyperglycemia (Acute Stress Response, Cushing Syndrome, Pheochromocytoma, Glucagonoma, Corticosteroid Therapy)

Decreased levels

Hemolytic anemia or other diseases with shortened red blood cell lifespan such as sickle cell disease and glucose- 6 – dehydrogenase deficiency, chronic blood loss, chronic renal failure.

CALCIUM (Ca) - TOTAL AND IONIZED CALCIUM

Reference Range

Total Ca: 8.6-10 mg/dL, 2.15-2.5 mmol/L
Ionized Ca: 4.64-5.28 mg/dL, 1.16-1.32 mmol/L

Clinical Implications

Increased levels (Hypercalcemia)

Hyperparathyroidism, Cancer with Parathyroid Hormone (PTH) – Producing Tumors (Metastatic Bone Cancers, Hodgkin Lymphoma, Leukemia And Non – Hodgkin Lymphoma), Paget Disease of the bone, Prolonged Immobilization, Milk-Alkali Syndrome, Excessive intake of Vitamin D, Milk, Antacids, Addison Disease, Granulomatous Infection (E.G., Sarcoidosis, Tuberculosis).

Decreased levels (Hypocalcemia)

Pseudo hypocalcemia caused By Low Albumin Levels, Hypoparathyroidism, Renal Failure, and Hyperphosphatemia Secondary to Renal Failure, Rickets, Vitamin D Deficiency, Osteomalacia, Malabsorption, Pancreatitis, Malnutrition, and Alkalosis.

SODIUM (Na)

Reference Range

135-145 meq/L

Clinical Implications

Increased levels (Hypernatremia)

Increased Sodium Intake (Dietary or IV), Decreased Sodium Loss (Cushing Syndrome, Hyperaldosteronism), and Excessive free body water loss (GI, Excessive Sweating, Extensive Burns, Diabetes Insipidus, and Osmotic Diuresis).

Decreased levels (Hyponatremia)

Decreased Sodium Intake (Deficient Dietary or IV Sodium), Increased Sodium Loss (Addison Disease, Diarrhea / Vomiting, Intraluminal bowel loss, Diuretic administration, Chronic Renal Insufficiency, Gastric Suctioning), Increased free body water (Excessive Oral Or IV Water Intake, Hyperglycemia, CHF, Peripheral Edema, Pleural Effusion, SIADH)

POTASSIUM (K)

Reference Range

3.6- 5.0 mEq/L

Clinical Implications

Increased levels (Hyperkalemia)

Excessive Dietary or IV Intake, Acute or Chronic Renal Failure, Addison disease, Hypoaldosteronism, Aldosterone – inhibiting diuretics (Spironolactone, Triamterene), Crush or Cell Damaging Injuries (Accidents, Burns, Surgery, Chemotherapy), Hemolysis, Acidosis, Dehydration.

Decreased levels (Hypokalemia)

Deficient dietary or IV Intake, Burns/Trauma/Surgery, Diarrhea/Vomiting/Sweating, Diuretics, Hyperaldosteronism, Cushing Syndrome, Licorice ingestion, Alkalosis, Glucose administration, CF.

PHOSPHATE (PO$_4$), PHOSPHOROUS (P)

Reference Range

3.0-4.5mg/dL , 0.97-1.45mmol/L

Clinical Implications

Increased levels

Renal Failure, Hypoparathyroidism, Acromegaly, Bone metastasis, Sarcoidosis, Hypocalcemia, Addison disease, Rhabdomyolysis, Healing fractures, HypervitaminosisD.

Decreased levels

Hyperparathyroidism, Hypercalcemia, Rickets, Malnutrition, Gram-Negative Sepsis, Hyperinsulinism, Alkalosis, IV Glucose administration (phosphorous follows glucose into cells), Starvation, Malabsorption syndrome, Hypomagnesemia, Chronic alcoholism, Vitamin D deficiency, Nasogastric suctioning, Vomiting.

TOTAL ALBUMIN

Reference Range

3.5-5 g/dL, 30-50 g/L

Increased levels

Dehydration

Decreased levels

Ascites, burns, Glomerulonephritis, Liver disease (hepatitis or cirrhosis) or acute inflammatory disease, Malabsorption syndrome (e.g., Crohn disease, Celiac disease or Whipple disease) and malnutrition.

TOTAL PROTEIN

Reference Range

6.4-8.3 g/dL: 64-83 g/L

Increased levels

Inflammation or Infections, such as Viral hepatitis B or C or HIV, Bone marrow disorders, such as Multiple Myeloma or Waldenstrom's disease.

Decreased levels

Bleeding, Liver disorder, Kidney disorder Such As Nephrotic disorder Or Glomerulonephritis, Malnutrition, Malabsorption conditions such as Celiac disease Or Inflammatory bowel disease, Extensive burns, Agammaglobulinemia, Inflammatory condition, and Delayed post recovery surgery.

BLOOD UREA NITROGEN (BUN)

Reference Range

5-20mg/dL, 1.8-7 mmol/L

Clinical Implications

Increased levels

Prerenal (Hypovolemia, Shock, Burns, Dehydration, CHF, Myocardial Infarction (MI), Gastrointestinal (GI) Bleeding, Excessive Protein Ingestion, Catabolism, Starvation or Sepsis), Renal (Renal Disease or Failure, Nephrotoxic drugs), Postrenal (Urethral obstruction from stones / Tumors/ Congenital Anomalies, Bladder outlet obstruction from Prostatic hypertrophy, Cancer, or Congenital Anomalies).

Decreased levels

Liver Failure, Acromegaly, Malnutrition, overhydration, Negative nitrogen balance, Syndrome of inappropriate secretion of antidiuretic hormone (SIADH), Pregnancy, Nephrotic Syndrome, Anabolic steroid use, Impaired Absorption (Celiac Disease).

CREATININE (SERUM CREATININE)

Reference Range

Female: 0.5-1.1 mg/dL, 44-97 µmol/L

Male: 0.6-1.2 mg/dL, 53-106 µmol/L

Clinical Implications

Increased levels

Impaired renal function (e.g., Glomerulonephritis, Pyelonephritis, Acute Tubular Necrosis, Urinary Tract Obstruction), Muscle Disease (Gigantism, Acromegaly), Rhabdomyolysis, Shock (Prolonged), Diabetic Nephropathy, CHF.

Decreased levels

Debilitation, Decreased muscle mass (e.g., Muscular Dystrophy, Myasthenia Gravis), Advanced and Severe liver disease, with age proportional to decrease in muscle mass.

References

1. Mahan, L.K., & Raymond, J.L. (Eds.). (2016). *Krause's food & the nutrition care process*, (14thed.). St.Louis, Missouri: Elsevier.
2. Width, M., & Reinhard, T., (Eds.). (2018).*The essential pocket guide for clinical nutrition*, (2nded.).India, New Delhi: Wolters Kluwer.

NON NUTRITIVE SWEETENERS

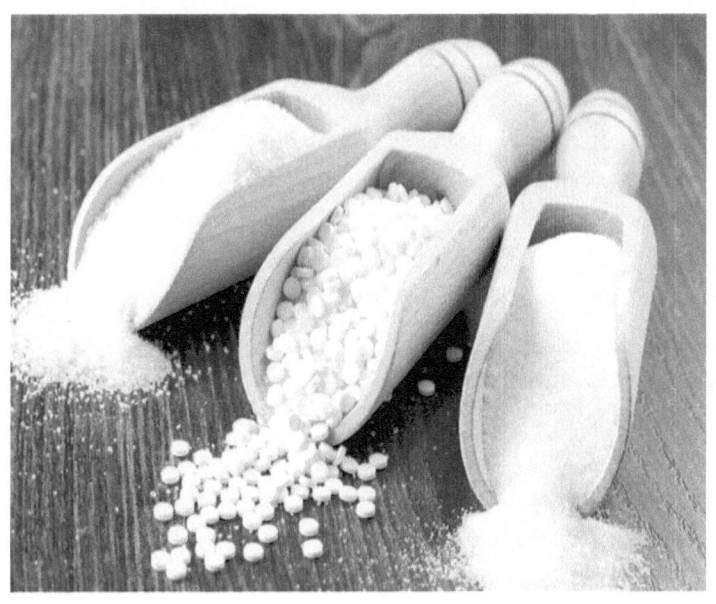

Non Nutritive Sweeteners (NNS) are generally regarded as sugar substitutes or sugar alternatives, they are many times sweeter than sugar but contribute only a few, to no calories when added to foods). / Artificial sweeteners./ Low- calorie sweeteners/ Intense sweeteners are the different names labeled for substances such as Sucralose, Aspartame, Acesulfame-K, Saccharin, Neotame, Stevia, recent additions to the list being Advantame and Swingle fruit extract. These products are generally added to jams, jellies, sweets, ice- creams, candy, pudding, soft drinks, baked foods, etc as they are claimed to be beneficial over nutritive sweeteners (sucrose, fructose, etc) which contribute calories and carbohydrates) that increases the risk for dental caries, obesity, pre-diabetes, type 2 diabetes and cardiovascular disease(3). These agents belong to different chemical classes giving a sweetness ranging from 300 – 13000 times sweeter than sucrose.NNS is regulated as a food additive and is generally recognized as safe (GRAS). Currently, 6 sweeteners are FDA-approved as food additives: Saccharin, Aspartame, Advantame, Acesulfame Potassium (Ace-K), Sucralose, Neotame whereas Stevia and Fruit Extract are GRAS. Foods containing polyols and/or no added sugars, within food labeling guidelines, can be labeled as sugar-free nutritive sweeteners. Polyols, a natural sweetener (also referred to as sugar alcohols) also add sweetness with less energy (2 kcal/g) and may reduce the risk for dental caries and when consumed on regular basis could cause osmotic diarrhea in children.

Unfortunately, there are minimal studies to depict the long-term use of NNS and associated health effects. Any sweet taste will induce an insulin response that results in blood glucose uptake by the tissues, but since artificial sweeteners will not lead to a rise in blood glucose, it will result in hypoglycemia and hence increased food intake (4). Long-term studies are required to confirm these findings.

Recent study shows that over-consumption can result in dysbiosis and metabolic abnormalities including glucose intolerance (2). Hence while prescribing an artificial sweetener, remember to check whether it is FDA approved and if it is within the Acceptable Daily Intake (ADI). It's important to choose NNS based on the type of diabetes and associated comorbidities.

Table 1 USFDA approved NNS

Sweetener	Regulatory Status	Examples of Brand Names Containing Sweetener	The multiplier of Sweetness Intensity Compared to Table Sugar (Sucrose)	Acceptable Daily Intake (ADI) (mg/ kg bw/day)	Number of Tabletop Sweetener Packets Equivalent to ADI*
Acesulfame Potassium (Ace-K)	Approved as a sweetener and flavor enhancer in foods generally (except in meat and poultry) 21 CFR 172.800	Sweet One® Sunett®	200 x	15	23
Advantame	Approved as a sweetener and flavor enhancer in foods generally (except in meat and poultry) 21 CFR 172.803		20,000 x	32.8	4,920
Aspartame	Approved as a sweetener and flavor enhancer in foods generally 21 CFR 172.804	Nutrasweet® Equal® Sugar Twin® Sugar-Free Gold®	200 x	50	75
Neotame	Approved as a sweetener and flavor enhancer in foods generally (except in meat and poultry) 21 CFR 172.829	Newtame®,	7,000-13,000 x	0.3	23 (sweetness intensity at 10,000 x sucrose)

Sweetener	Regulatory Status	Examples of Brand Names Containing Sweetener	The multiplier of Sweetness Intensity Compared to Table Sugar (Sucrose)	Acceptable Daily Intake (ADI) (mg/ kg bw/day)	Number of Tabletop Sweetener Packets Equivalent to ADI*
Saccharin	Approved as a sweetener only in certain special dietary foods and as an additive used for certain technological purposes 21 CFR 180.37	Sweet and Low® Sweet Twin® Sweet'N Low® Necta Sweet® Sugar-Free ®	200-700 x	15	45 (sweetness intensity at 400 x sucrose)
Siraitiagrosvenorii Swingle (Luo Han Guo) fruit extracts (SGFE)	SFGE containing 25%, 45% or 55% Mogroside V is the subject of GRAS notices for specific conditions of use GRAS Notice Inventory	Nectresse® Monk Fruit in the Raw® PureLo®	100-250 x	NS***	ND
Certain high purity steviol glycosides purified from the leaves of Stevia rebaudiana(Bertoni) Bertoni	≥95% pure glycosides Subject of GRAS notices for specific conditions of use GRAS Notice Inventory	Truvia® PureVia® Enliten® BeStevia® Sunova® Steviocal® GaiaStevia®	200-400 x	4**	9 (sweetness intensity at 300 x sucrose)
Sucralose	Approved as a sweetener in foods generally 21 CFR 172.831	Splenda® Sugar-free Natura®	600 x	5	23

* Number of Tabletop Sweetener Packets a 60 kgs (132 pounds) person would need to consume to reach the ADI. Calculations assume a packet of high-intensity sweetener is as sweet as two teaspoons of sugar.

**ADI established by the Joint FAO/WHO Expert Committee on Food Additives (JECFA)

*** NS means not specified. A numerical ADI may not be deemed necessary for several reasons, including evidence of the ingredient's safety at levels well above the amounts needed to achieve the desired effect (e.g., as a sweetener) in food.

Table 2 NNS Safety in Pregnancy and Lactation

NNS	SAFETY
Acesulphame K	Avoid, and in renal/hyperkalemic
Aspartame	Moderation-U
Saccharin	Avoid
Neotame	Not Determined
Sucralose	Safe

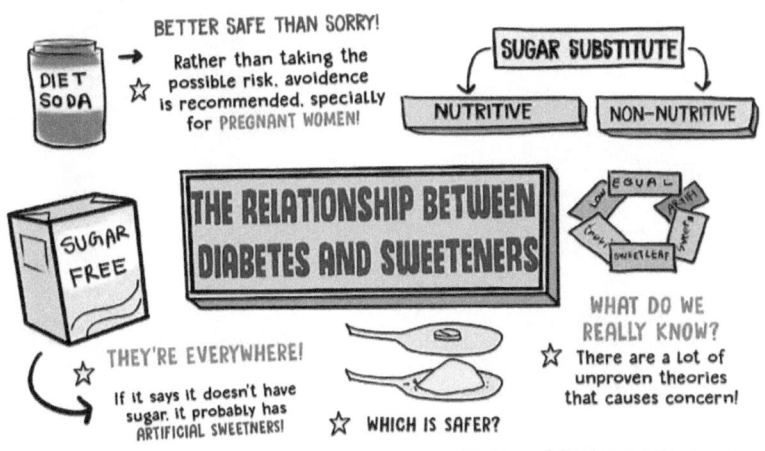

References

1. High-intensity sweetener. (n.d). Retrieved from https://www.fda.gov/Food/IngredientsPackagingLabeling/FoodAdditivesIngredients/ucm397725.htm
2. Suez, J.,Korem, T.,Zeevi, D.,Zilberman-Schapira, G.,Thaiss, C. A., Maza, O., Israeli, D., Zmora, N.,Gilad, S., Weinberger, A., Kuperman, Y., Harmelin, A., Kolodkin-Gal, I., Shapiro, H., Halpern, Z., Segal, E.,&Elinav.E.(2014).*Artificial sweeteners induce glucose intolerance by altering the gut microbiota,514,* 181–1 86.
3. Fitch, C., & Keim, K. S (2012). Position of the Academy of Nutrition and Dietetics: use of nutritive and non-nutritive sweeteners, *Journal of Academy of Nutrition Diet, 112*(8), 1279.
4. Kirtida, R.T. (2011).Sugar substitutes: Health controversy over perceived benefits, *Journal of Pharmacol Pharmacother, 2*(4): 236–243.
5. *Clinical Dietetics Manual, Indian Dietetic Association,* 2011, 1(3): 25.

EDUCATING THE PUBLIC ON

Educating the public on the Bajaj's Rule of 80 to live healthily up to 80

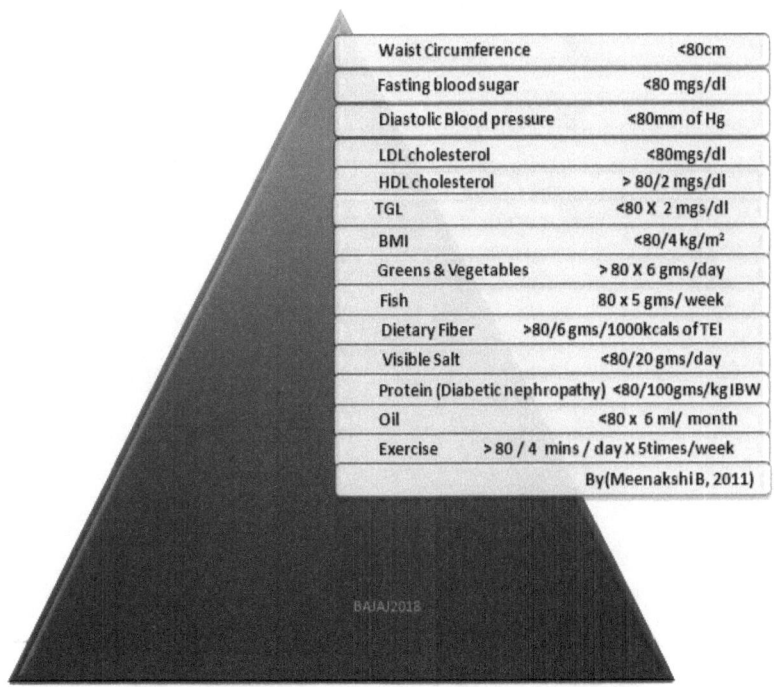

Waist Circumference	<80cm
Fasting blood sugar	<80 mgs/dl
Diastolic Blood pressure	<80mm of Hg
LDL cholesterol	<80mgs/dl
HDL cholesterol	> 80/2 mgs/dl
TGL	<80 X 2 mgs/dl
BMI	<80/4 kg/m²
Greens & Vegetables	> 80 X 6 gms/day
Fish	80 x 5 gms/week
Dietary Fiber	>80/6 gms/1000kcals of TEI
Visible Salt	<80/20 gms/day
Protein (Diabetic nephropathy)	<80/100gms/kg IBW
Oil	<80 x 6 ml/ month
Exercise	> 80 / 4 mins / day X 5times/week
	By(Meenakshi B, 2011)

BAJAJ2018

Citation: Bajaj.M, "BAJAJ'S RULE OF 80", Diet Metrics, 2018